S0-DOO-168

Amelia

Enjoyed our hours before
class — and happy to
learn This made it to
6TH & 48TH. Best of luck!

Richard

Mortal Men

Mortal Men

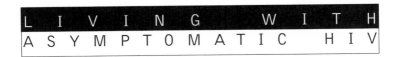

LIVING WITH
ASYMPTOMATIC HIV

Richard MacIntyre

RUTGERS UNIVERSITY PRESS
New Brunswick, New Jersey, and London

Library of Congress Cataloging-in-Publication Data

MacIntyre, Richard, 1952–
Mortal men : living with asymptomatic HIV / Richard MacIntyre.
p. cm.
Includes bibliographical references and index.
ISBN 0-8135-2596-9 (alk. paper)
1. HIV-positive persons—Interviews. 2. Gay men—Interviews. I. Title.
RC607.A26M389 1999
362.1'969792—dc21   98–8501
CIP

British Cataloging-in-Publication data for this book is available
from the British Library

Copyright © 1999 by Richard MacIntyre
All rights reserved
No part of this book may be reproduced or utilized in any form or by any means,
electronic or mechanical, or by any information storage and retrieval system, without written permission from the publisher. Please contact Rutgers University
Press, 100 Joyce Kilmer Avenue, Piscataway, NJ 08854–8099. The only exception
to this prohibition is "fair use" as defined by U.S. copyright law.

Manufactured in the United States of America

For Helen Miramontes

CONTENTS

FOREWORD

"Everyone I love is dying or dead. This is personal. I'm not being scientific. My world is destroyed. . . . My past is disappearing before my eyes. . . . There's no witness to my life."

—Dick

Marcel Proust once observed that great experiences do not inevitably make people either wiser or more observant—that, for example, a mediocre writer, asked to describe a significant event such as fighting in the trenches during World War I, will still reduce that event to banality and cliché. For Proust, the power of successful narrative depends on the transforming vision of the writer, not on the quality of the event itself. Yet *Mortal Men* illustrates how a deep personal and communal crisis may elicit the most profound observation among those it affects. Granted, the people Richard MacIntyre interviews are not writers. But as they seek out—and find—language adequate to their experience, we are reminded how wisdom may grow through the telling of one's own story. Although AIDS, tragically, provides the historical and personal crises at the heart of *Mortal Men*, the figures who emerge from these pages seem far from tragic. This narrative as a whole centers on survival, on those living with long-term asymptomatic HIV. Yet as readers we are never allowed to forget that courage and compassion, ruth and renewal are the price and gift of survival—that survival in the context of loss may lead to a unique and even eloquent reengagement of the self.

In the course of reading *Mortal Men*, one is initially struck by how much the speakers—and the interviewer himself—share in common. All are urban gay men whose sexual liberation either coincided with the arrival of AIDS or predated it by less than a decade. All are articulate, educated members of a relatively exclusive, highly eroticized social world, a world that consisted of lovers, former tricks and boyfriends, would-be sexual conquests, and friends who shared common assumptions about the body. After years of cultural and political activism and communal commitment to gay pride, all had taken their lives and their world as won—wrested from a heterosexist and broadly homophobic culture. The arrival of AIDS severely tested such assumptions. These speakers all found themselves and their world suddenly under terrible siege, a siege that required them to renegotiate their contracts with life and, consequently, with their own mortality.

Literary critics and social scientists have frequently noted that during the first decade of the crisis, AIDS tended to impose its own grid on individual experience. As MacIntyre asks his interviewees how AIDS first entered and affected their lives, each individual narrative moves toward a personal past, centered in the 1980s, and involving a sexuality and sense of self brought up short by the fact of plague. And it does come to each in what initially appears to be patterns. First one reads about a new, "gay" cancer in the press—the gay press, because the national media were largely ignoring the crisis; then friends are touched by it; and soon someone one knows dies. There follows the agonizing decision about whether to be tested for HIV, and this during a time when, in Dick's words, a positive test result translated as "You're dead"—and your death will be horrible.

Even when these interviews were made, in the early 1990s before hope was provided by new "drug cocktails," gay men were still living in what author Andrew Holleran has called "The Fear": that period from the late 1980s on when AIDS was no longer a distant abstraction. MacIntyre's research occurred when AIDS was peaking in the gay community; when countless lives were devastated by the deaths of friends, lovers, coworkers; when it seemed everyone was caught up in his own mortality; when death seemed inevitable, one's situation uncertain, and progress in fighting AIDS nonexistent.

Thus deciding to be tested for HIV, and being found positive, are necessarily central to each person's narrative. What occasions this decision is, in part, a reflection of character as well as of individual circumstance; it embodies a critical self-encounter and so becomes as fascinating and distinct as is each speaker himself. Of course, other central questions inevitably follow such a diagnosis. Whom can I trust with this knowledge? Should I inform my future sexual partners? Will I monitor my T cells? Will I embrace AZT or a holistic alternative? Confronting HIV and the tough personal questions that come along with it reveals people's fragility and their strengths. It throws into relief each person's unique beliefs about life and death; his relation to his past as centered in family, community, or ideology; and his relation to his possibly greatly truncated future. In these speakers' stories, HIV crystallizes and compresses those issues that, for most people, take a full lifetime to sort through.

What is fascinating about MacIntyre's subjects is that at the height of the epidemic none of them equated diagnosis with death, either psychologically or physically. Even though friends and lovers have died, while the community they knew and its way of life have largely disappeared, each of these speakers is still asymptomatic and has been so for years. Thus their histories anticipate the current medical situation in which people on drug cocktails, having previously faced their probable early mortality, are forced to rethink their relation to their own futures—futures that might now actually become realities. And here MacIntyre's narrators may prove trustworthy guides: despite their fears, virtually all of them have made decisions about their futures that, however tenuously, assume continuance: they have completed residencies and advanced degrees, they have constructed new lives in new places, and they have made fresh commitments to love.

HIV positive himself, Richard MacIntyre is uniquely positioned to elicit and interpret these stories. As a gay urban medical professional who shared in the sexual liberation and in the community of his subjects, he is able to bring multiple perspectives to bear on their narratives. His nursing training and its painful application in the age of AIDS have prepared him to be empathetic and understanding; his sexual frankness encourages his narrators to be candid about their own most intimate and personal experiences. Not only are most of the speakers his friends or acquaintances who could trust him to share many of their values, but the interviews themselves were originally conducted as part of an academic project, which encouraged his speakers to be thoughtful and reflective.

Yet initially these multiple perspectives and voices do not seem to fit neatly together. The tonality of the early interviews feels jarring, almost disjointed, as whimsical sexual dialogue comes up against the professional language of medicine and treatment. However, out of this fascinating divergence of language and issues, MacIntyre emerges as a mediating presence who can listen empathetically to those friends who are afraid of finding themselves in the ranks of the ill. Some struggle with the symbolic meaning of T cells, which is often psychologically more overdetermined than its actual medical significance; others see themselves transformed from instruments of pleasure to vessels of death and contamination, and they must cope with body images that have been devastated.

Thus MacIntyre's own story of his personal and professional development is extremely important. Largely recounted in chapter 2, but punctuating the interviews throughout, his experience enables us to contextualize the other stories and to appreciate their differences. For this reason, the narrative structure of *Mortal Men* differs radically from most other AIDS memoirs, which have largely focused on the deaths of lovers (Paul Monette's *Borrowed Time;* Mark Doty's *Heaven's Coast*) or on individual searches for a cure (Paul Sergio's *One Boy at War*) or for a cause (Gabriel Rotello's *Sexual Ecology*). Like Abraham Verghese's *My Own Country*, the study of AIDS and its impact on a single community from a doctor's perspective, this nurse's account is structurally a "frame tale," where one memoir or story occasions and encourages the telling of others. This technique gives the book its richly multivocal tonality.

Of the many themes at the heart of *Mortal Men*, certainly identity and survival rank as paramount. For all the speakers, sexuality in the era of gay liberation has served as a conduit for the discovery of a new self that could be free; for some, HIV reveals the fragility that underlies this achieved identity. Yet ultimately the self and the communal awareness of these speakers seem deepened, enriched, and even ennobled by confrontation with the reality of HIV in their lives. At times MacIntyre's friends reflect on their situations with humor bordering on camp: "What I miss most about sex in the old days . . . was being called a slut and taking it as a compliment" (Matthew). At others, ruminating on mortality leads his subjects to insight: "The lines that so naturally and so quickly extend out from our own narratives about ourselves, that extend out into the future—all of those lines, all of a sudden, were chopped . . . [and] ended in an abrupt chasm. . . . A certain amount of our lives is based on decisions way down the road. . . . I don't think about it much anymore. It's harder sometimes. It's harder to do" (Gabe).

Making sense of life, loss, and survival, of debilitating illness, of the terrible testing of one's community—these are, after all, great issues, and many of MacIntyre's subjects have achieved great and vibrant wisdom in coming to terms with them. Certainly Dick's fear that there would be no witness to his life is assuaged by the power of his own narrative. His voice, like those of the other speakers—always articulate, frequently passionate, vulnerable, funny, and profound—makes his story, and theirs, unforgettable.

—*Stephen Lacey*
Cornell College, Iowa

ACKNOWLEDGMENTS

During the Middle Ages Dante inveighed against popes who coveted the power of emperors; in literary retaliation Dante hung several of them upside down in a hellpit for eternity. Today it is the pope's position that is coveted, not by the emperor, but by leading researchers in the health sciences. Recently, one of my colleagues characterized a particular group of researchers as "running around like a bunch of redhats, wanting to be pope." And she knew what she was talking about. She is one of nursing's most respected leaders, a member of the President's Commission on AIDS, a faculty member at the University of California at San Francisco, and a volunteer for the vaccine trials. This book is for her, Helen Miramontes, a mother who knows and a colleague who cares.

Most professional education is about preparation for the future, and this is perhaps as it should be. However, in 1988, after losing two lovers and testing positive for HIV myself, I could not contemplate five more years of graduate school geared toward some future academic career that I might never see. I am therefore especially grateful that I had the opportunity to work with professors such as Anne Davis, Marylin Dodd, and Patricia Benner at the University of California, San Francisco—professors who believed that doctoral work in nursing might be something valuable in and of itself—without reference to where it might lead.

I am only one among thousands of practicing nurses who are grateful to Patricia Benner's pioneering work on excellence in nursing practice.

Rather than employing traditional models and measures, her work focused on the stories and conversations that nurses shared with each other about their patients. Through those stories modern nursing is beginning to discover its collective identity and its potential for excellence. Whereas much of the university persists in dividing the world up into discrete and measurable bits and pieces, Benner encourages her students to start stitching it back together again—however tentatively—by searching for the meanings and understandings that people develop in response to suffering and difficulty. I could not have started the intellectual and moral journey that resulted in this book if Patricia Benner had not first cleared a path. As a dissertation committee chair she provided the critical intellectual stimulation and supportive validation I needed to complete my Ph.D. As a friend and mentor she opened doors that allowed me to keep writing.

Stephen Lacey was my first mentor. As a gay nineteen-year-old at the University of California, Santa Barbara, I was deeply interested in what made people tick. I soon tired of rats and switched my major from psychology to English literature. Lacey taught Shakespeare, Proust, Dante, and Marlow from a Freudian perspective—but he never let Freud or theory stand in front of the texts he was teaching. The nursing profession has a great, largely untapped resource in our colleagues from the humanities. Over the several years it took my predissertation interpretative papers to evolve into this book, Lacey offered numerous thoughtful critiques of my thinking and writing.

Much of the work involved in turning my dissertation into a readable book occurred 250 miles north of the Arctic circle at the northernmost university in the world—the University of Tromsø in Norway. Several Norwegian colleagues and friends either provided explicit feedback on drafts or helped in a myriad of ways to make our stay in Norway both pleasant and productive. I thank Per Grøholt and Margorie Parker of the Norwegian Center for Leadership Development in Oslo; Inger Margrethe-Holter, chief nurse at the Rikshospitalet in Oslo; and Professor Kari Martinsen and the nursing faculty at ASV in Tromsø. Especially helpful critiques were offered by nursing faculty, Jarle Grumstad, and Fulbright professors Per Kristian Roghell (nursing) and Rachael Stewart (minority literature).

I am also grateful to the William J. Fulbright Foundation for funding my year abroad and to Jean Olsen, director of the American-Norwegian Fulbright Office, for helping to make the 1996–1997 academic year the most exhilarating in my career. And none of this would have been possible had not Samuel Merritt College extended my sabbatical leave after my postdoctoral fellowship at the International Center for HIV/AIDS Research, a World Health Organization Affiliate at the University of California, San Francisco. I am especially grateful to the center's director, William Holzemer, who gave me an opportunity to complete a review of the literature in HIV and alternative medicine before commencing my work on the book in Norway.

I am particularly thankful to my editor, Martha Heller, not only for her superb editing, but also for her boundless energy, infectious humor, and unwavering belief in this project. I am also deeply appreciative to those in my extended family who took the time to read and critique the manuscript—Timothy Volmer, Eric Archibique, Martin Karlow, Karlien Bach, Claudine Lacey, and Mary Rothleitner, my mother-in-law.

And to the heavenly hosts who saw fit to bless me with a partner, Robert Head—a man who followed me to the end of the earth, who softened every discouraged moment, and who shared every bright one, who critiqued, edited, and talked me through every muddled thought— I am eternally indebted.

Finally, to the HIV-positive men who shared their stories and their lives with me—you are so beautiful. Thank you.

Mortal Men

| 1 |

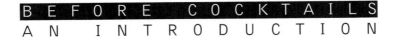

B E F O R E   C O C K T A I L S
A N   I N T R O D U C T I O N

In 1995 the war against HIV took yet another turn. News flashes announced that something on the magnitude of a paradigm shift had happened to medical thinking about the virus associated with AIDS. Previously, scientists had thought there was an extremely variable and often very long latent period when HIV simply hid in the body without causing much damage. Such thinking occurred because many people who tested positive for the HIV antibody were not showing serious symptoms or were taking a long time to develop them. Most of these "asymptomatics" had fewer T-helper cells, or CD4 lymphocytes, understood to be the primary target of HIV.[1] But they were not getting sick. Today thousands of people have been living with HIV for well over a decade without developing AIDS.

The "latency" idea reigned in scientific circles from 1984 until 1995, when influential virologists concluded that there was no latent period in HIV infection after all.[2] HIV was replicating not only in the CD4 cells but also in other white blood cells and in the lymphatic tissue. Those who remained relatively asymptomatic year after year were actually quite sick, their bodies engaged in what scientists called a "pitched battle" with the virus from day one. People who managed to remain asymptomatic were pumping out new CD4 cells almost as fast as HIV was killing them. But the virus was not sleeping.

I first read that HIV infection had never been latent in an AIDS update sponsored by a pharmaceutical company and published in the Journal of the Association of Nurses in AIDS Care.[3] I had been living in San Francisco's gay Castro district for twenty-one years. I had been living with asymptomatic HIV for eleven years, having tested positive for HIV in 1985. In 1993 I completed a Ph.D. in nursing on asymptomatic HIV infection. The concept of latent HIV infection, dismissed with great fanfare in 1995, was actually never central to the conversations about HIV that I was hearing in San Francisco's Castro district. Almost none of the physicians, researchers, or patients I knew ever talked about HIV as if it were latent. For years medical doctors had been attributing our problems with shingles, thrush, rashes, fatigue—even the fungus growing under our toenails—to HIV infection. And if the virus was latent, what was causing so many of our T cells to disappear? Sleeping viruses don't kill T cells. Perhaps the pharmaceutical company's "update" was simply intended to build up a feeling for the tremendous breakthrough that its new antiviral drugs represented. But the twist on our historical understanding of HIV infection troubled me.

The antivirals that were introduced in 1995 brought more hope into the struggle against AIDS than all of the previous AIDS therapies combined. Some people with full-blown AIDS were literally getting up off their deathbeds with the new treatments. But for those of us with asymptomatic infection, reactions were mixed. Whereas many people with asymptomatic HIV jumped at the chance to fight the virus with the new drugs, others remained as skeptical about medical intervention as they had been from the beginning of the epidemic.

In the early 1990s a number of opinions existed about whether antiviral medications such as AZT were good or bad. Back then a number of informed and well-educated gay men were rejecting both the laboratory tests used to monitor HIV infection and the drugs used to fight it. Many of these men gave what seemed to be valid reasons for rejecting the help offered by the medical establishment. Antiviral medications were often toxic and of questionable value. Frequently, physicians were more pessimistic than their patients. The blood tests used to monitor HIV infection were presumably to help one decide when to take the toxic, possibly useless drugs, but nobody really knew what the right time was. Unfortunately science will probably never know how many lives were prolonged and how many were shortened by the early treatments for HIV and AIDS.[4]

Despite these understandable reasons for not seeking medical attention, others seemed to stake out ideological positions in response to what I thought were basically biomedical or clinical questions. Otherwise intelligent people conflated theories of government conspiracy and corporate greed into explanations for why AIDS existed in the first place and why there was still no cure. As a nurse and an HIV-positive gay man, I was perplexed by this and decided to focus my doctoral studies around the issue.

People infected with HIV have either embraced, rejected, or felt ambivalent about each new product and pronouncement from the medical industry. Making appropriate decisions about technological advances has become increasingly complex in our society. Technology creates new norms, new economic pressures, and new understandings that change the way we think about our lives. The bulk of our AIDS activists have spent the last fifteen years advocating for new medical interventions, and their persistence is finally paying off. But there has always been another more hidden story, a story of sometimes wearied skepticism.

Gay men with asymptomatic HIV infection had reason to be skeptical. Historically, the medical profession was only a very recent "friend." Prior to 1974 medicine still defined gay people as mentally ill. Rather than the pinnacle of a liberating twentieth-century enlightenment, the medical profession seemed to some gay men yet another expression of simultaneously oppressive and empty modern values.

There were big problems with the medical response to AIDS, even where no ill will toward its victims was intended. I had sat in conference after conference where well-meaning doctors and public health officials flatly declared that HIV was 100 percent fatal. How do they know? I wondered. And why do they say what they can't possibly know? A few AIDS leaders continue to pontificate similar nonsense to the press. In 1997 one leading AIDS doctor in San Francisco announced that he knew what happened to people who did not take their antiviral medications. "They die," he was quoted as saying in one newspaper. And perhaps his patients do, but many have lived with HIV for fourteen or more years without ever having taken antiviral drugs.

The statistics projecting when people with asymptomatic HIV would sicken and die didn't pan out either.[5] The "average" time of surviving with HIV increased one year almost every year after academics started predicting it. Some people with HIV understood that the official public health predictions were dead wrong, yet still found it possible to trust their own private physicians. But for others, the whole system was suspect.

People with asymptomatic HIV were asked to fight a virus they could not see and a disease they could not feel. They were asked to change sexual practices that often formed the core of their identities. They were asked to trust a profession and an industry infused with the politics of power and profit. Yet with little else in the way of help or hope, this was often the best thing to do.

Rational arguments have been made for and against almost every advance in AIDS care, whether the issue is taking a blood test, taking a drug, or taking early retirement. This book is not so much about the pros and cons of various treatment options as it is about how a group of gay men confronted and lived with those options in the early 1990s. Since that time the blood tests and the drugs have changed, but the major issues surrounding treatment and monitoring decisions have not. Today the treatments are better, but the stakes are just as high. This narrative, almost an autobiographical history of gay men with asymptomatic HIV infection, shows how a small group of bright and articulate gay men experienced the ministrations of their doctors and the pronouncements of the press. It describes how people with asymptomatic HIV infection took up or resisted the way friends and community were understanding HIV. It reveals how identities were constructed during an era of liberation and reconstructed during an era of death.

Monitoring HIV Infection: A Short History

By 1996 physicians had three basic blood tests with which to diagnose and monitor HIV infection. The first, commonly known as the "HIV test," had been widely available since 1985. At that time "the test" was much more controversial than it is today. Several articles in gay publications urged people not to take it. In 1985 there were no medical treatments for HIV. We sent people who were suffering from AIDS to the hospital and treated their strange infections or cancers as best we could, but there were no treatments for people who simply tested positive for "the virus." On top of that, those who did test positive faced enormous social problems. HIV-positive adults were getting fired from their jobs and losing their medical insurance, and HIV-positive children were being barred from schools. In one study, more than 50 percent of nursing students felt they should be allowed to refuse to care for people with HIV.[6] In such a milieu it is no wonder that the test was controversial.

Those who did decide to take the test were told that, unlike other antibodies, the HIV antibody offered no defense against the new virus. Rather, antibodies against HIV meant something new. Instead of protecting us against the new virus, this particular antibody meant that the entire immune system would eventually be overwhelmed by it. Experts estimated that about 50 percent of the gay men in San Francisco were infected with HIV.

Within a few years several things changed and the gay media started advocating the HIV test. Anonymous test sites became available in several states, which protected people against some of the social fallout from testing positive. The eventual inclusion of HIV/AIDS in the Americans with Disabilities Act helped as well. In addition, new medical tests and drugs became available for monitoring and treating HIV infection. Campaigns for HIV testing were launched throughout the nation, which further reduced resistance to HIV testing.

After 1987 people who tested positive for the HIV antibody had to decide whether to take advantage of the second medical test, T cells. These cells are an integral part of the immune system. A count of the T cells made possible a general picture of the damage inflicted on the immune system. Publications such as *Science* and the *National Geographic* carefully explained the central role T cells play in mediating our immune response to foreign proteins. Because of extremely promiscuous sexual practices, many urban gay men had been in contact with record numbers of foreign proteins. T cells, specifically the T-helper cells (or CD4 cells), are one of the body's major defenses against foreign proteins, and they were slipping away. Diagrams and photographs showing HIV attacking a CD4 cell were inscribed indelibly on our minds. Most HIV-positive gay men had CD4 cell counts under 800, about one-half to two-thirds of the normal number.[7] Those suffering from full-blown AIDS usually had CD4 counts under 100 or 200.

By 1988 HIV disease was restaged according to the T-cell count. More than 500 T cells generally meant that one would not develop AIDS within the next three years. Between 200 and 500 was understood as a gray zone where minor problems with thrush or hairy leukoplakia were not uncommon.[8] Fewer than 200 used to mean

AIDS-related complex (ARC); today fewer than 200 CD4 cells constitutes an AIDS diagnosis. However, the numbers reflected general probability patterns in the population, not absolute predictions. Some
people developed symptoms even with 700 T cells. Others walked
around with counts under 50 and almost no symptoms at all.

The availability of new ways to monitor HIV infection meant that
HIV-positive patients and their physicians had to make new decisions.
Those who chose to monitor their T cells faced a number of additional
challenges, not the least of which was determining what those numbers
meant in terms of their own lives. People facing that decision between
1987 and 1995 had to decide whether or when to start taking antiviral
medications, whether to begin one or a number of alternative treatments, and whether lifestyle changes might be appropriate. Some
patients and physicians had strong ideas about what all the numbers
meant. There still wasn't much solid scientific research, however, especially for those with more than 500 T cells and those without symptoms. From the beginning many gay men were forced to draw their own
conclusions about their T-cell counts. Yet without the guiding benefit of
science, some decisions about monitoring, treatment, and lifestyle issues
were not always consistent or easily understood.

The third test became widely available in 1996. This test made it possible for medical science to estimate the strength of the viral enemy circulating in the blood. In addition to calculating the damage inflicted on
the immune system, the third test could measure the number of viral
particles circulating in the blood, or "viral load." By stimulating viral
particles into exponential reproduction, a lab technician could amass a
"load" of particles large enough to measure. Critics argue that the new
test doesn't really "count" or "weigh" the virus, but very high viral loads
do correlate with morbidity.

Viral load results are harder for people to interpret because they are
reported in logs rather than normal numbers. In 1996 results of 30,000
and 50,000 were indistinguishable to physicians, but patients often
attribute meanings to small shifts that physicians would call insignifi-
cant.[9] This is not unlike tumor markers for cancer. A normal range for
tumor markers after treatment for breast cancer is less than 36, but
many patients react emotionally to increases or decreases within that
range, even when intellectually they know better. Much more importantly, viral load testing changed the standard for what counts as
"healthy" for people with HIV. When virologists abandoned their ideas

about latency, the concept of a "healthy" HIV-positive person was also largely abandoned. Today much of the medical industry thinks that the decision to forgo or postpone antiviral treatment is like fighting a deadly battle without the benefit of bullets.

What constitutes "health" for a person with asymptomatic HIV will continue to change in response to technological advances and economic pressures. The health of a person with HIV used to be divided into stages of severity based on T-cell counts, but after 1996 the stages were replaced with a singular understanding—infection with a killer virus. A high T-cell count used to be very good news for people with HIV. Today many believe that the only possible good news is an "undetectable" viral load. Yet even undetectable isn't really low enough because HIV is understood to be replicating in the lymphatic system, where it cannot be measured.

Treating HIV Infection: A Short History

In addition to blood tests, the medical industry also developed new drugs. AZT, the first approved drug for fighting HIV infection, became available in 1987. AZT wasn't actually "developed" to fight HIV. It was an old cancer drug that had been discarded as too toxic. AZT works against HIV by blocking reverse transcriptase, an enzyme necessary for DNA synthesis. The most common side effect is bone marrow depletion, which in turn causes anemia. Results from the studies that investigated the efficacy of AZT were mixed. Like the early days of radiation and chemotherapy for cancer, it was not always clear whether the treatment was slowing death down or speeding it up.

By 1990 there was only one approved drug for HIV and it seemed as toxic for people as it was for the virus. The lack of progress in the development of medications besides AZT (which was exorbitantly priced) produced a good deal of outrage in the community and in part spawned the ACT-UP (AIDS Coalition to Unleash Power) movement. Activists were successful in pressuring the pharmaceutical company that owned AZT into reducing the price. Activists were also influential in getting the Food and Drug Administration (FDA) to streamline its approval process for new drugs. On this issue they found common ground with the same pharmaceutical companies they were otherwise fighting, and several new and improved reverse transcriptase inhibitors (ddI, ddC, D4T, 3TC) became available. Prior to 1996 most patients and physicians used the T-cell count to help decide whether to start antiviral therapy.

In 1995 a new class of drugs was introduced—the protease inhibitors. These also work by inhibiting DNA synthesis, specifically by preventing protease from being added to the DNA chain. The protease inhibitors continue to look promising when used in combination with the reverse transcriptase inhibitors. Early experience with combination therapy shows both greater efficacy against the virus and fewer side effects. Marked reductions in viral load and even sustained increases in CD4 cells are not uncommon in patients taking the new "AIDS cocktail." But there are serious drawbacks. Side effects can include serious increases in serum cholesterol and diabetes-like symptoms. In addition, when used alone, the protease inhibitors quickly lose their effectiveness. Furthermore, people who count their T cells, take their antivirals, and measure their viral loads have to contend with the possibility of developing mutant strains of HIV that become unresponsive to the drugs. Fears of creating new mutant strains of HIV surfaced at the 1996 AIDS Conference in Vancouver, where some public health officials envisioned supervised therapy for those who did not take their medication properly.

Advocates for pharmaceutical intervention tend to call the antiviral drugs "reverse transcriptase inhibitors" or "protease inhibitors." Opponents of the blanket use of antivirals for HIV infection call the drugs "DNA chain terminators." Both are correct. The terms *reverse transcriptase inhibitor* and *protease inhibitor* make it easier to visualize the medication inhibiting something that the virus needs. Opponents, notably Peter Duesberg, point out that both reverse transcriptase and protease are essential building blocks for DNA, in every strand, in every species.[10]

Many are impressed at the significant clinical improvement in very sick people, but some clinicians remain unconvinced at the advisability of putting long-term asymptomatics on the powerful new drugs. In 1997 the *Wall Street Journal* reported that the life spans of people living with AIDS had been increasing before the new drugs and technologies became available.[11] This should not be surprising. Thomas McKeown reported a similar story about tuberculosis in England: "Streptomycin, developed in 1947, was the first effective treatment [for tuberculosis], but by this time mortality from the disease had fallen to a small fraction of its level during 1848–1854. Streptomycin lowered the death rate from tuberculosis in England and Wales by about 50 percent, but its contribution to the decrease in the death rate since the early nineteenth century was only about 3 percent."[12] We often forget that nature takes a shape, even without our interventions. Health professionals are sometimes tempted to take credit for natural phenomena and for every HIV-positive person alive today. But some people with HIV are not taking antiviral medications, good though they are for others.

Those who resist medical monitoring and antiviral treatment have to contend with mounting pressure to conform to normative standards and expectations. This has been true from the beginning. Despite all the carefully constructed language about personal choice at the anonymous test site centers and the rhetoric about informed consent, gay men who continue to resist medical monitoring and antiviral intervention are often labeled as being "in denial" both by health professionals and by other gay men. Pregnant women with HIV face even greater pressures. But the new drugs and blood tests force everyone to make new decisions. Whether one ultimately decides to take advantage of the new technology (and if so, when and for how long) depends on how one has come to understand HIV/AIDS and how others in one's life and community understand it. One's HIV antibody status, T-cell counts, and viral loads are personal concerns and are consequently interpreted within a context of particular beliefs, experiences, and relationships. In addition, the trust that people with HIV have in the health care system affects the way they understand HIV, and this varies from complete trust, to fragile trust, to overt distrust and fear.

Preventing Progression from HIV to AIDS

Michael Callen was one AIDS activist who did not trust that the health care system was asking the right questions. Callen's own question was straightforward: "Why were some people with AIDS living longer than others?"[13] Dr. Richard Rothenberg, an AIDS researcher at the Centers for Disease Control (CDC), deemed Callen's question unanswerable: "A prospective study would of course be best. But even to do a good retrospective study, we'd need to review the charts of about 5,000 people with AIDS. We've also been hoisted by our own petard of confidentiality. I'm afraid we've just missed the boat on this one. The best study of long-term AIDS survival hasn't been done, and probably will never be done. The logistics are insurmountable."[14]

Rothenberg's conclusion would have been even more pessimistic had the question of long-term survival been applied to people with asymptomatic HIV infection rather than AIDS. Although the confidentiality of one's HIV status is specially protected in some states, AIDS has never commanded more confidentiality than any other illness. If Rothenberg found the logistics for studying AIDS survival insurmountable, studying HIV survival would be even worse. Rothenberg's conclusion was based on his conception of what constitutes good science, but medical science is not the only legitimate way to develop knowledge about health. Callen, a man who lived with the serious AIDS-defining problems from 1982 to 1994, continued to explore his question by interviewing people who had survived a diagnosis of full-blown AIDS for three years or longer—double the average length of survival at the time. His work reflected the determination of a journalist: tracking down leads, talking to the key players (patients, physicians, policymakers, researchers) and reading all he could on the subject. For daring to suggest that his own history of passive anal intercourse with over two thousand men had damaged his health, several AIDS activists labeled Callen "homophobic." And for daring to suggest that HIV was not the only causative factor in the development of AIDS, some medical experts labeled Callen "demented." Yet to my mind, Callen produced the most interesting work to date on surviving AIDS.[15]

For researchers, the progression of HIV to AIDS is much harder to study than the progression of AIDS to death. The specific mechanisms involved in end-stage AIDS are easier to identify than the mechanisms of asymptomatic HIV infection. How to prevent HIV from progressing to AIDS has always been one of the most important questions for people living with HIV, but this question has been too unwieldy for any of our health disciplines to warrant a comprehensive and sustained research effort. Thousands of people in the United States and western Europe have been living with relatively asymptomatic HIV infection for more than ten years. Many of these have been living with HIV for fourteen to twenty years, some without antiviral treatment.[16] But despite these numbers and the millions of dollars spent by the public health and biomedical research establishment on AIDS, efforts to explain why some people with HIV live long healthy lives while others die quickly have been paltry at best.

Public health officials have been understandably occupied with preventing the spread of HIV. The bulk of research in psychology and the social sciences has focused on high-risk behaviors associated with the spread of HIV in the "general" population. Almost none of the research projects undertaken at the well-funded but somewhat misnamed Center for AIDS Prevention Studies (CAPS) has been concerned with preventing the progression of HIV infection to AIDS. Psychoneuroimmunological studies have tried to identify factors that would predict progression to AIDS, but basic descriptive and epidemiological research on survival has not been a national priority. Nursing has tended to mirror the concerns of the other health disciplines and has focused either on prevention of the spread of the virus or on the physical and psychosocial care of the seriously ill.

Biomedicine pursued antiviral and antimicrobial agents and, to a lesser degree, chemical means to bolster the immune system. The need to treat identifiable illness and postpone death in the seriously ill overshadowed the need to prevent healthy people with HIV from developing AIDS. What efforts there were stemmed from treatments designed for those suffering from serious illnesses. A few drugs developed for people with advanced immune disorders were tested for their preventive potential in relatively healthy people. Septra, for example, is used to prevent the development of pneumocystis pneumonia in people with fewer than 200 T cells. In addition, antivirals are sometimes given to people with 500 or more T cells, but to date there is no scientific evidence to indicate that these early interventions do more good than harm.

Asymptomatic HIV-positive gay men have found themselves at the intersection of a number of competing approaches to health and illness, including Western biomedicine, traditional ethnomedicines, and a variety of complementary and alternative modalities. At the center of this competition are theories about the immune system, not only the mechanics of its defenses against microbes and cancers, but also its relationship to psychological, lifestyle, and social issues. In addition to seeing their physicians, people in the HIV-positive community are also visiting acupuncturists, ingesting herbs, and joining gyms. Gay men, especially those with asymptomatic HIV infection, are seeking out a variety of approaches to treat it. As with other diseases, those who stay relatively healthy have much more freedom to choose or refuse treatment. Serious symptoms tend to force people into existing structures for care and treatment where dominant cultural understandings prevail.

But the freedom from symptoms and the freedom to refuse culturally sanctioned therapies for asymptomatic HIV infection create a degree of ambiguity, ambivalence, and even hostility among some asymptomatics. This is especially true in such cities as San Francisco and New York, where health and illness are understood from a variety of different perspectives. Family, friends, and physicians often push different treatments and approaches and sometimes react to the patient's choices with ambivalence rather than support.

None of this is to imply a level playing field for the holistic and biomedical positions. Western medicine defined AIDS and discovered HIV. Western biomedical understandings of disease dominated public discussions of HIV and AIDS, shaped the structure of HIV and AIDS services and research, and became the credo of almost every major AIDS organization. A century ago Robert Koch and Claude Bernard argued about the relative role microorganisms play in human diseases. Koch focused on microbes, whereas Bernard argued that medicine must pay attention to the human terrain that microbes (which are everywhere) invade.

Some gay men with asymptomatic HIV heeded Bernard's warning against the "single minded fervor of the microbe hunters," especially since the early drugs used to fight HIV were often both ineffective and dangerous. Some of these men focused on stress reduction, drug and alcohol use, nutrition, exercise, and meditation.[17] Others developed fantasies about being able to control their HIV and T-cell counts with right living and right thinking, becoming examples of the "blame-the-victim" critique that Western medicine has leveled against the holistic health movement.

However, the vast majority of gay men embraced Western medicine. We grew up in a culture informed by the notion that diseases are caused by single, identifiable, and measurable agents. People who accepted the dominant, medical construction of AIDS understood that the illness was caused by a chance encounter with a virus. The religious and political right, however, construed the epidemic as the scourge of an angry God or the consequences of an immoral agent—"the wages of sin is death" approach.[18]

A more holistic approach to AIDS would have included psychosocial and behavioral issues, such as the rampant promiscuity, alcoholism, and drug use in the gay community, but the battle lines had been drawn. The religious and political right proclaimed our guilt and picketed our funeral services, while the biomedical establishment insisted that the virus was morally neutral and would infect whomever it could. The cause of AIDS became a black-or-white issue: a blame-the-victim mentality parading as personal responsibility or a blame-the-virus mentality parading as hard science. Given those choices, it's no surprise that most people with HIV felt more comfortable with the latter.

When the scientific establishment did address psychosocial and behavioral issues, it was almost always within a viral framework. Researchers seemed to conclude that studying behavioral issues that were not directly related to contracting HIV (and the social structures that sustained them) might be construed as being homophobic or blaming the victim. The viral framework had the distinct advantage of appearing objective, amoral, and nonjudgmental, and most humanists and academics opted for the "HIV is the cause of AIDS" equation.[19]

Over time, however, as people accumulated more experience living with HIV, the assumption that the virus held all the cards seemed unduly pessimistic and disempowering. In addition to pursuing traditional holistic approaches to sustaining health, such as nutrition, detoxification, exercise, acupuncture, and herbs, many gay men started reappraising specific social structures and practices in their community. The gay liberation movement had forced gay men out of the closet and into a world where they were compelled to develop new identities and ways of understanding themselves. That all this gay liberation and gay identity construction took place within a largely hostile and homophobic culture immersed in its own narcissism and hedonism has not been fully appreciated. A sexuality and sensuality that had been repressed and restrained throughout adolescence (and for eons) suddenly exploded. Not all of the practices that develop around liberation movements are valorous or healthy. Some take a serious toll. But the notion that behaviors associated with gay liberation contributed to the decimation of gay men's immune systems continues to be both psychologically untenable and economically unprofitable. It is far more comforting for patients and far more profitable for the medical industry to attribute the entire epidemic to a chance encounter with a virus.[20]

Yet the notion that lifestyle might affect who remains asymptomatic and who progresses to AIDS has been part of the conversation among gay men with asymptomatic HIV for well over a decade. This hasn't been an easy conversation. The major party boys did seem to drop dead first, but lots of us knew men who had lived cleaner lives but were already dead. Thus, questions about the effect that drugs, alcohol, stress, depression, and promiscuity might have on disease progression persist in the gay community, both consciously and subliminally. These questions aren't simply due to unresolved feelings of guilt, self-loathing, or internalized homophobia. Although emotions often accompany such questions, rational minds will pose them independently. But the questions have been hard to answer.

Far more radical questions are being posed today, particularly concerning "bareback" sex (anal intercourse without a condom). How risky is bareback sex between two gay men with asymptomatic HIV? How risky is it if these two men are monogamous or mostly monogamous? Theoretically (and officially), HIV-positive people should avoid bareback sex to avoid further exposure and a possible increase in viral burden. Some men with asymptomatic HIV buy this, but others reject this theory with a variety of arguments, including a risk-benefit type of analysis. A still more radical group is preaching a version of the pope's dictum that sex is a natural gift from God and that therefore gay men should practice it naturally—that is, bareback. Today even some HIV-negative men are advocating bareback sex on the (to my mind dubious) argument that the safe-sex movement is a Gestapo tactic designed to create "SEX PANIC," which ultimately interferes with real, intimate contact between gay men. The sex-panic group thinks that the safe-sex movement can be more dangerous than HIV. Others, who often note the deaths of numerous friends and lovers, get almost spastic with horror and moral indignation at the mere suggestion of a gay man having sex with an unprotected penis. This group would also revise the pope's position on penises and make all sex without a condom a sin for those not intending to conceive a child.

Science does not know how people with asymptomatic HIV can prevent their conditions from turning into AIDS. Even the fine print on the pharmaceutical advertisements admits that we don't know whether antiviral medications will prolong the asymptomatic period. We also don't know whether reducing stress will prolong the asymptomatic period, whether abstinence from drugs and alcohol will prolong the asymptomatic period, whether eating right, exercising right, meditating right will prolong it. After all this time, we don't even know whether condom use between HIV-positive partners will prolong life. Yet even though science has not answered these questions definitively, people with asymptomatic HIV answer them every day, within the contexts of their own lives, experiences, and beliefs.

Whereas most of the top AIDS researchers give lip service to the existence of "cofactors," the role that these and other non-HIV-related factors might play in the progression of HIV to AIDS has not been seriously investigated. For example, Duesberg's hypothesis that drug use (particularly poppers) plays a significant role in the development of AIDS is not consistent with the research priorities developed by the National Institutes of Health (NIH).[21] The war against AIDS has a single strategy: seek out the virus wherever it may be lurking and kill it. But the single-minded focus on the virus is not confined to the medical establishment. When Rotello suggested that two thousand or more sexual partners per decade may not be a biologically sustainable norm in any community, many outspoken gays accused him of being homophobic.[22] Nonetheless, the views of dissident and often marginalized academics and community leaders who suggest that other factors besides the virus should be considered are seriously entertained by many gay men living with HIV. Michel Foucault's work on the relationship between scientific truths and the structures of power that develop and sustain them has inspired serious thinkers to reconsider the biomedical construction of HIV/AIDS.[23] Those who have lived with asymptomatic HIV infection over the last ten to fifteen years have had to chart their courses between these larger cultural arguments about health, microbes, and disease.

The Project

As a holistically minded nurse, I had always been deeply ambivalent about biomedical science and AIDS. In 1985 I spoke at a Mobilization Against AIDS rally at United Nations Plaza in San Francisco and flatly declared that biomedical science would never find a cure for AIDS. In my view, too many activists suffered from the delusion that the medical industry could still produce silver bullets for every health problem. I believed that the primary cause of AIDS was a virus. I still do. What I did not believe was that destruction of the virus should focus all of our research efforts and all of our hopes. At the same time I did not understand the positions taken by several of my friends. Some of my friends were forgoing the laboratory tests used to monitor the progression of HIV and rejecting even the possibility that pharmaceuticals might eventually prove helpful.

My first obligation, both as a nurse and as a researcher, was to appreciate the various ways people in my community were confronting HIV. God knows, the topic was discussed everywhere. People were talking about HIV infection between sets at the gym, over coffee in cafés, and in the middle of sidewalks in the Village and the Castro. The National Institutes of Health always sang in unison, even before the advent of the AIDS czars: people with HIV should be regularly monitored and, with their physician's recommendation, should take the drugs that received official approval. However, the voices of asymptomatic HIV-positive gay men in my own community were cacophonous variations on a dominant theme—"Am I really sick?"

The ramifications of this question reverberate in each of the stories that follow. Some argue that we should think of HIV as a chronic condition. They call for regular medical monitoring and efforts to safeguard our immune systems—whether we feel healthy or not. Their hopes are pinned on faster scientific advances, and some of their agenda has been translated into new public policy. Of course, there are as many different ideas about how to safeguard the immune system as there are hedonistic pleasures to destroy it.

Others argue against medical monitoring. They warn us to avoid the "sick identity" like the plague—think positive; laugh; indulge in pleasures aimed at affirming life. To be consumed with "Should I do this? Should I do that?" is to have lost life anyway.

Another group tries to achieve a sort of balance between these approaches. These folks try to define themselves as healthy, but at the same time they work to safeguard their immune systems by making as many lifestyle changes as they possibly can—again, whether they feel healthy or not. They count their T cells, consume vast quantities of health care (holistic, allopathic, or both), and try to have the "right" attitude about it all. My own voice joins those calling for balance, but trying to find a balance among biomedical, sociopolitical, and holistic concerns produces more questions than it does answers.

The stories in this book recount how several gay men came to take the HIV test and how it subsequently changed their sexuality, their social relationships, and their health practices. Competing positions on all these issues emerged in the community. Some call for an end to promiscuity. Others defend it. Many wrestle with feelings of contamination. Some simply do the best they can to cope with the accumulated grief from losing so many friends and loved ones. Acceptance or rejection by family, friends, and colleagues varies from person to person, as do opinions about appropriate medical monitoring and treatment. Although terribly unscientific, personal experiences are precisely the context in which people come to understand HIV infection and the ways in which it might be treated, monitored, or ignored.

In addition to my own, this work includes ten stories that were selected from among the hundreds that I heard during the late 1980s and early 1990s. These stories formed the basis for my doctoral research and were derived primarily from in-depth interviews I conducted during 1990 and 1991.[24] Each participant in this study had known or suspected his HIV-positive status for several years. These were not traditional research subjects in that I did not contact them through a clinic or an advertisement in a newspaper. These were men I knew. Some of them were close friends. Others were men I had met at the gym, a bar, or a sex club. They were all between twenty-five and forty-five. A handful of people is never truly representative of a community, yet these men constituted the particular community in which I lived and the community I, to a large extent, lost.

In the early 1990s viral load testing and the AIDS cocktail were not available. Back then the standard approach was to monitor HIV by counting T cells and to treat it by prescribing reverse transcriptase inhibitors (AZT, ddI, DDC). Today the new tests and new treatments are finally creating some real hope. People with HIV are living longer now. But the new approach is also creating new complexities and pressures that bear some striking similarities to those that people with asymptomatic HIV have been facing from the beginning—defining health while making sense of new and changing lab values, managing sex and drugs in a culture of indulgence and liberation, considering treatment options within the context of community norms and individual beliefs, caring for loved ones (with or without HIV) who may be fearful, needy, sick, or dying.

The stories told here are those that most engaged me as a nurse, a researcher, and a gay man who is himself HIV positive. They reveal a group of gay men living with conflicting theories, metaphors, and pressures in their community. They show how dominant understandings of health and disease are resisted and how they are taken up. They tell how a group of people in my community came to experience mortality, medicine, and health in an era of sex, drugs, and T cells. Yesterday's struggles are set down here in the hope that our humanity might be preserved and our future endowed with the insights that we developed in response to death.

This book reflects the observations, thinking, and feelings of a man who lived in the eye of the storm for twenty-five years. The work is, of course, limited by my own perspective and experiences, but nurses are experienced readers of live human texts, and it is from the multiple perspectives of nurse, friend, and lover that this work proceeds. I hope it will offer new insights and possibilities to others coping with serious illnesses and to those who must construct new meanings in the midst of death and the technologies engineered to prevent it.

| 2 |

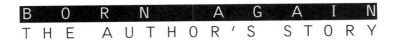

BORN AGAIN
THE AUTHOR'S STORY

Christmas 1971 ended with an ultimatum.

"Your mother and I," my father announced, "can no longer finance the Devil's work in your life. You have three choices: (a) move back home, live in a Christian atmosphere, and go to San Jose State; (b) transfer to Oral Roberts University in Tulsa, Oklahoma; or (c) show evidence of a renewed relationship with Jesus Christ."

I made my decision on the Greyhound bus whisking me back to Santa Barbara. It happened just south of Gilroy where U.S. 101 streaks through a rolling landscape of green and gold. Option "A" was out of the question. I saw myself as an eleven-year-old boy pulling weeds, sweeping cement, and reorganizing the woodpile. I was thankful for the weeds, the dirt, and the chaos that disturbed the woodpile and created Saturday chores. I selected my chores strategically in order to avoid the man in the garage, an ominous dark force we called "Daddy." At any moment I might be summoned to learn something practical, to fetch tools, to absorb abuse. Hateful hours were spent watching incomprehensible activities under the hood of a car. If I failed to learn something—and I learned absolutely nothing during those hours—I was being obstinate. That boy would have given anything to please the man, but it wasn't in him.

Sunday afternoons were for throwing balls in the backyard. I threw like a girl, and Daddy was sure that I did it on purpose. He didn't get it.

He knew I was a mama's boy but somehow failed to comprehend that mama's boys never piss off their six-foot, four-inch, 200-pound fathers on purpose.

A spare-the-rod-spoil-the-child Baptist, Daddy managed his deep depressive nature with shouting, swearing, and smacking. His sovereignty in the household had been established by God, and Daddy's need for control knew no bounds. Daddy was a navy man who thought his house was a ship and his family a crew. Humiliation was a constant companion of those who lived with him. While pulling weeds, I used to calculate the hours and minutes that separated me from what would someday become my life. My brothers did the same. During these calculations an inner, yet distant voice always promised me that things would get better after I left home, after I finished high school.

The time was now. That inner voice I had heard as a child was my own. I was finished with Christian family life in San Jose. The Greyhound crested a hill, and California's central valley stretched south like a magic carpet, rolling toward a new life. I briefly considered option "B."

Two years earlier I had seriously thought about going to Oral Roberts University. I had started playing the piano for a gospel group that sang at the little Pentecostal church in the neighborhood. The rest of the family attended the Baptist church, but a tiny degree of flexibility made it possible for me to substitute an evening Pentecostal service for the Baptist one. I would have done anything to avoid spending time with Daddy, but I actually enjoyed the Pentecostal service. A few months later my mother had started attending a Tuesday morning prayer meeting at the same church. One evening when Daddy was working late, Mother asked me to go to a revival meeting at the Pentecostal church. "Don't tell me you've started speaking in tongues," I said. She didn't respond. At the end of the service, while the organ was playing, I walked up to the altar with several other folks. There I prayed that God would heal me of being gay. I prayed myself into a frenzy and was rewarded with the Gift of Tongues and the Baptism of the Holy Ghost, becoming yet another one of God's charismatic queers.

Daddy was not yet a charismatic. At the time he was not at all interested in paying for private tuition at a Pentecostal college in Oklahoma. Option "B" would certainly be preferable to the hellish Christian home life in San Jose, but I had already changed too much. Santa Barbara had seduced me with nude beaches, sex, and other illicit pleasures, and I had just discovered Sigmund Freud and Marcel Proust. Oklahoma had no beaches, and Oral Roberts would be no place to study Freud or Proust. As for option "C," I could have pretended a renewed relationship with Jesus Christ, but Jesus still meant too much to me to fake it.

I wasn't athletic or handsome or mechanically inclined. Over time it would take hundreds of men to convince me that I was attractive. It would take countless bodybuilders writhing on their stomachs to re-kindle the sense of masculinity Daddy had all but extinguished. The only thing I had always been good at was school. Despite my father's proclamations that I would never amount to anything, I quietly told myself that my brains would earn me enough money to pay someone else to fix the car, the washing machine, and the toaster. My brain was fully engaged. I knew how to take multiple-choice tests. The answer was clear: "D"—none of the above.

Nursing

When the Greyhound pulled into Santa Barbara, this nineteen-year-old pregay, post–Jesus-freak homosexual had a plan. Do the winter term. Then quit school. Get a job. Buy a stereo. Begin a life. The job would have to pay at least $3.00 an hour and give me one thing I had never had—control over my hair.

During the winter term 1972, I met Phil, a screaming queen in his midtwenties. He was sunbathing in the dunes near the university. Those dunes were as hot as the sands in the seventh circle of Dante's *Inferno*. As a sodomite, my feet were condemned to an endless, tiring trek, while my libido, ignited by the proximity of forbidden passions, blazed. Phil was Italian, with flashing green eyes, perfect proportions, and an all-over tan that glistened under a coat of dark brown hair. The first few times were fun, but he was far too nelly to hold my sexual interest.[1]

Phil worked as an orderly at a local hospital but carried himself like a professional. He paid close attention to his appearance—uniform neatly pressed, hair and nails trimmed, and just enough foundation and mascara to cause a twitter in the nurses' lounge.

Phil assured me I could con my way into a job at his hospital. It paid $3.25 to start, and long hair was no problem. Lots of the orderlies fastened their ponytails off their collars with one of those leather thongs and a stick. The traditional route to the gender-neutral "hospital attendant" position was six months' work in a convalescent hospital, but that paid only $2.10 per hour and the work would be terminally boring for this nineteen-year-old. "Don't do that," Phil advised. "You're way smarter than most of the people they hire. Just say you can do TPRs [temperature, pulse, and respiration], blood pressures, S&As [sugar and acetone tests on urine], bed baths, transfers from wheelchair to bed, bed to wheelchair, and I&Os [figuring of fluid intake and output]. And tell them you have experience with feeders and foleys. They'll teach you how to put catheters into pee-pees, so you don't need to say you can do that."

The job sounded perfectly awful. I had never liked science, snails, or puppy dog tails. The very idea of the orthopedic traction equipment on Phil's unit scared me. I never, ever, wanted to work in a hospital. But I didn't have any other bright ideas.

Not being very comfortable with lying, I concocted an elaborate story to get the job. My application would say I had graduated from high school a year early and moved to Germany to work as an orderly in Munich. Whereas I had studied German for five years, I had never actually been to Germany. Surely they wouldn't call Germany to check a reference for an orderly position. A German job would also account for my deficiencies in medical terminology. It was a perfect story.

I put on my Sunday best and trotted through interviews with three separate women, each in full nurse drag, each sitting behind neat desks in ground floor offices, far away from the nearest patient. The last one gave me a test. After reading a few lines about a patient situation, I was required to put the information into a simulated medical record. My junior high school math skills helped me successfully plot the TPR and blood pressure on the graphic sheet, but it was my decision not to enter this information into my "nurse's notes" that got me the job.

"You were probably wondering why you had this interview with me," said a rather butch Mrs. Fullwood. "People have to interview with me because I can tell who's had experience and who hasn't." As a pit formed in my stomach, I tried to effect a look somewhere between deadpan and dumb jock. "And I can tell by your charting that you have experience. People who haven't worked in acute hospitals will always chart the TPR in the nursing notes." She blathered on for a while before issuing instructions about where and when to report for orientation. I was elated. That one successful lie was to change the course of my entire life.

During my orientation I once ventured onto Phil's unit. From halfway down a long hospital corridor, I was greeted with an out-stretched arm, hand fluttering wildly at the wrist, and a "Hel-loooow!"

about an octave higher than the charge nurse could have produced. Sensing my discomfort, his fluttering hand settled on his hip while his eyebrows arched, his head cocked, and his lips pursed: "So, darling, how does it feel to be Miss Nurse?"

For a few weeks I stayed at Phil's apartment, where he sometimes served as a surrogate parent. His penchant for "wrecking them" prefigured the in-your-face Queer Nation politics of the 1990s. I followed suit. Bleached-blond hair and a smart jumpsuit gave me the confidence I needed to wreck them with my outrageousness in the shopping malls. But this quickly proved tiresome. I didn't give a rat's ass for shopping malls or suburban queens.

Santa Barbara always sported at least three nude beaches, and except for one aborted attempt at school, I divided my time the next year among the beach, the hospital, and sex. I knew that I wasn't headed anywhere, and that bothered me. Some of my friends were artists of one variety or another. A handful were becoming lawyers or accountants, but most were doing very little. At twenty-one, my biggest fear was turning thirty without knowing what I wanted to be when I grew up. Then I saw a little flyer outlining a registered nursing curriculum at the junior college. I couldn't help but notice that I had already completed most of the required nonnursing courses. Would it be worth two years out of my life to be guaranteed a decent income?

I had not fallen in love with nursing during the course of my hospital duties. I was under no illusion that I wanted to be a nurse. I believed the nursing program would amount to subtracting two years from my life. But being a registered nurse would be preferable to being an orderly, and the probability that I would still be working as an orderly two years hence was sobering. After graduation I thought I might work as a psych nurse for a while. Perhaps that would lead to my being a psychologist. If I started right away, I would graduate by age twenty-three. I could start worrying about what to do with my life then. With an R.N., I could even move to San Francisco, which, like Santa Barbara, was light years away from San Jose.

By summer of 1975 I had taken the board exam for registered nursing. After five lovely years in Santa Barbara it was time to move on. I packed my belongings and my new Siamese kitten into my VW bug, and we were off to San Francisco.

During my first few years in San Francisco I lived with my ex-lover, Bruce, a man I had met in Santa Barbara in 1972. We rented a Victorian flat in the Castro and decorated it with vintage garage sale items from the 1930s and 1940s. We stripped the living room fireplace with paint remover and dental tools and painted the walls a deep forest green. The walls sported old deco prints in period frames. Even the toilet seat was oak. It was antimodern, antififties, and, perhaps unconsciously, antiparent. We ate brunch at the Island restaurant, a hippie joint where even the waiters looked organic, with their long hair, patched jeans, and glazed eyes. Fashion was changing a few blocks away on Castro Street, and acid rock was giving way to speed disco. But the Island restaurant, Hamburger Mary's, and The Stud still breathed the spirit of the counterculture, and it was righteous.

Santa Barbara had been like training wheels, both personally and professionally. I started working the 3 to 11:30 P.M. shift—perfect for gay life in San Francisco. I could hit the bars after work and the gym in the morning and still have enough time left over to take some courses toward my baccalaureate degree. Within six months San Francisco transformed a carefree, long-haired beachboy into a hard-bodied urban clone.

San Francisco was also where I finally had to take on the sobering responsibilities associated with being a registered nurse. My ward cared for adolescent patients with cancer, cystic fibrosis, asthma, or orthopedic problems. We also took care of adult patients when the other medical and surgical units were full. The pace was fast, but the real challenge for me was to slow down. Individuals are hard to recognize when medications and procedures are delivered at breakneck speeds, and I often worked way too fast to appreciate the unique needs of those entrusted to my care. But occasionally I slowed down enough to get the story and in the process was able to give something more than standard care.

One evening Mrs. Porter, a lovely, bright, and articulate woman in her midseventies, gave me a very troubled look when I handed her a consent form for the cerebral arteriogram she was scheduled for the next morning.[2] Mrs. Porter had experienced some blackouts and was in the hospital for tests. About ten months earlier she had had a cerebral arteriogram for the same problem, but it had been negative. Mrs. Porter didn't want to go through it again and was very clear that she didn't care if her blackouts were due to a brain tumor or a small stroke. There was nothing to do if she had suffered a small stroke, and she had no intention of undergoing either chemotherapy or surgery. Mrs. Porter was not depressed. She was not despondent. She told me that she had lived a good life and didn't want it to end with chemo or brain surgery. And she was crystal clear about not needing to know whether she had cancer. She simply wanted to live until she got sick and died, and she did not want to undergo another cerebral arteriogram. Whereas Mrs. Porter did not need or want a diagnosis, she was troubled because her doctor did. She was from a generation where women deferred to men and everyone deferred to doctors.

This was my first major experience with "patient advocacy." Mrs. Porter was both intelligent and rational, and my job was to help empower her to make her own decisions. I told her to think of her physician as she would anyone else she might hire. He was there to give expert recommendations and to perform work if hired for the job. I argued that physicians should have no more claim to our bodies than lawyers would have to our lawsuits or mechanics would have to our cars. My frank advice could have easily spelled trouble, so I burdened the patient by requesting that she refuse the test with her own reasons and without reference to my comments as her evening nurse. Nurses were expected to get consent forms signed and support physicians' decisions, not contradict them. Mrs. Porter signed out the next morning against medical advice. I felt privileged to have been her nurse.

Another evening Mrs. Jefferson, the licensed vocational nurse (LVN) on my team, came into a room where I was reinforcing a dressing on a back surgery patient. Mrs. Jefferson had about twenty-five years of experience and was the most competent LVN on the ward.

"I know you're busy, Mr. MacIntyre. But just as soon as you can you better take a look at Mrs. Faircloth in room 516." She remained motionless until I was finished, making it quite clear I was to follow her, immediately if possible.

"You know I wouldn't bother you, and it may be nothing," she continued as we walked briskly down the long hall, "but Mrs. Faircloth is having a spell and she's hyperventilating. She said that the last time she had a spell like this she had a respiratory arrest and they had to call a Code Blue."

"Jesus," I thought silently. The last thing I needed was for some nut with low back pain to psych herself into dying. I remembered that her response to the stool softener I had given her an hour earlier was way off the wall. "God, I sure hope this helps," she had said with a bizarre sense of urgency. Ordinarily I would have explained that it took stool softeners a few days to make a difference. Ordinarily I would have asked her a few more questions. But I had several patients just back from major surgery, three of whom were not stable, and a ton of intravenous (IV) antibiotics and blood to hang. In addition, the girl whose acute asthmatic attack we had just stabilized worsened after the resident rammed a needle into her wrist for blood gases we didn't need. I didn't have a scintilla of extra energy for this woman and had shrugged off her emotion with slightly veiled contempt.

She must have been taking sixty breaths a minute. Her hands were clenched, her color was pallid, and her skin was clammy. Fortunately, a very simple intervention calmed her down. I told her to open her palms and breathe with me. I breathed rapidly for a while and then gradually slowed the pace. When her fists would start to clench, I would insist that she open them. Then I noticed a paraphrased edition of the Bible that was popular in the fundamentalist and Pentecostal communities I had once known so well. I asked Mrs. Jefferson to breathe with the patient for the next ten minutes while I checked on my bleeding back patient and gave some meds.

When I came back she was fine. An hour later when things were calmer, I went back into the room. To establish some rapport, I told her I had noticed her Bible and asked if she was a Christian. She said that she tried to be a Christian, but wasn't a very good one. She belonged to a Pentecostal church. I knew her world. Fits could come from only one of two possible sources.

"Oh, praise God," I said. "I am a Christian, too. Tell me, sister," I demanded, using all the male and professional authority I could summon. "Which is it? Are you plagued with a demon, or is God punishing you?"

I was fully prepared to conduct a brief exorcism, if needed, to keep her from freaking out. I didn't know whether I believed in demons, but I believed in getting rid of any demon that might be causing such an uproar on my shift. Fortunately, an exorcism was not required because God was punishing her. Although I was afraid that some of the words I spewed at her would stick in my throat, or that I would burst out laughing, I pulled it off with conviction. The other nurses didn't know her world or her language. The hospital chaplain, should one have been available, would probably not have known it either. My speech went something like this: "A minister once told me that the Devil's favorite lie was to say that God was angry with us. God almost never punishes

His children. He loves His children. If He sent Jesus down to die on the cross for all the sins of mankind, why would He pick out your measly little life for punishment? What kind of a witness for the Lord Jesus Christ can you be lying here in this bed? What kind of a wife or mother can you be here in the hospital? God loves you more than that. It is the Devil who is trying to separate you from God's love."

"Oh, thank you," the woman said. "I think you're right."

"What does your heart say? Is your spirit bearing witness to God's love?" I asked with a warm smile.

Three minutes later, after a prayer and a hug, I sped off to check the other patients and finish up my work. When I came back to work the next day, the woman had been discharged. I knew I had done the right thing, both as a nurse and as an estranged member of her spiritual community, but I couldn't share the story with anyone. Colleagues and friends alike would die laughing. I was a hell-raising homosexual, not a preacher man.

Had I stayed with that job, I would now have enough money to retire. But I decided to quit one night after having spent a very successful shift managing IVs. I'd been on the job just over three years. I was the only regular R.N. for thirty patients, eleven of whom had IVs. In those days we didn't hook each IV to machines with sensors and computers. Those machines were only for blood. So when we had to give an antibiotic IV, we clamped off the main liter-sized glass bottle, diluted the medication in a smaller plastic chamber that dangled below the main bottle, and ran it in. The trick was timing. We had to get back into the patient's room and open up the main bottle within two minutes or so after the medication was finished. Otherwise the IV might clot off, necessitating another stick for the patient and at least fifteen minutes of precious time. At the end of my shift I was really proud of myself. I had managed to get through eight and a half hours without losing one IV.

By the time I had changed into my bar clothes, I realized that nobody would ever know or care about my feat. If I became more efficient, the hospital would learn to count on me for more of the same. This was not a career; it was a job. I thought my recently completed baccalaureate degree should be good for something, so I took a job at what turned out to be a very disreputable vocational school. After a quick rise to the top of this nefarious organization, my colleagues and I closed it down. I spent the next three years working as a hospital nursing supervisor and completing a master's degree in nursing administration. I finished the master's degree in 1982 and started teaching again, this time in a bac-calaureate nursing program at Samuel Merritt College. The college had advertised for med-surg and mental health faculty, but my first assign-ment was teaching the management and health policy courses. It was a place that would stimulate my thinking and professional growth for the next fifteen years.

Love and Loss: Steve

These were the innocent years of liberation and indulgence when Eros taught us to celebrate sexuality and establish relationships. An old photo captured me, two ex-lovers, a recent fling, and my new lover all giggling hysterically at a mechanical bear. Confetti and birthday hats from my twenty-fifth birthday party dated the event as 1977. I had an old T-shirt that lamented, "So many men; so little time," and little did we know how true it was. Five years later the god of death arrived and taught us compassion and how to love through grief.

During 1977 I met two men who would change my life forever—my third lover, Steve, and my best friend, Gabe. Steve was my lover from 1977 until 1983. He had been a Rhodes scholar and student body vice president at a midwestern university before receiving his law degree at NYU. He was a quadruple Taurus who loved plants, cats, and classical music. He was sophisticated, handsome, and charming—160 pounds of muscle packed into a five-foot, eight-inch frame covered with dark, tanned skin and straight, sable fur. Within weeks after meeting, we had fallen head over heels in love. I flew to New York to meet him for a hon-eymoon. He whisked me from La Guardia Airport to a friend's East Side penthouse, where he barbecued shell steaks on a deck dominated by ficus trees and the New York skyline.

The next day we took the Long Island Railroad to Sayville, a cab to the dock, and a ferry to Fire Island Pines. A quarter of a mile wide and thirty miles long, Fire Island is a kind of sandbar to Long Island. One side looks out onto the bay and the southern coast of Long Island and the other onto the Atlantic Ocean. There are no roads and no cars. Dur-ing the summer months of the 1970s this island paradise must have included some straights and lesbians, but I noticed only a few deer and several hundred gay men.

For the first time in my life I was so much in love that I barely noticed all the other men. During the day the white sand beach provided a perfect backdrop for Steve's dark brown muscles. During one extraordinary night we walked along the beach, the sky splattered with stars and the ocean flooded with light from a full moon. When we stopped and sank into each other's eyes, my bones gave up a long-held secret: I had loved this man for an eternity.

Soon I found myself hopelessly in love and just as hopelessly unhappy. After a few weeks we had lots of commitment but little intimacy. A year later we moved to a beautiful home in the Oakland hills with a lush garden on a sun-drenched patio. We had four adorable cats. But I needed more than commitment. It took more than five years to satisfy myself that I could stick with a relationship through thick and thin, that I wasn't as fickle as most queens. But after five years I knew we had too much history for our relationship ever to improve, and I was finally able to end it. In 1983 I moved back across the bay to San Francisco. Until I could find my own place, I stayed with my best friend, Gabe.

Gabe was also a bright, East Coast boy with an impeccable sense of style and grace. At six foot, four inches tall and with lats as wide as an angel's wings, Gabe was also drop-dead gorgeous. But there the similarities between lover and best friend ended. Gabe was the smartest man I knew, intellectually and emotionally. He was an ABD (all but dissertation) from Stanford in English literature and supported himself as a writer. He published several books, most of them on dance, and wrote a few TV documentaries. One was narrated by Gene Kelly and another by Mikhail Baryshnikov, and a third was nominated for an Emmy. Gabe never made a fortune, but he enjoyed his work enormously. He was a big man in the big leagues and as sexually prolific as any professional athlete or rock star.

We talked about everything, as best friends are wont to do. At one point I was probably whining about turning thirty, getting divorced, and needing parental support, when Gabe suggested that I might be pushing my parents away rather than the other way around. (I was already somewhat reconnected with my parents. Over the years Mother and Dad were to meet all my lovers and Gabe.) He was probably right. I was creating at least some of the distance. So in late 1982 I invited both of them to lunch in Berkeley. I told them I didn't know how much or how little of my life they wanted to share; that I was very much in love, but that I needed to break up with Steve; that I didn't want to hear Bible verses. I also told them that gay men had started dying of a new disease that might be sexually transmitted. I told them that it was no time to be getting divorced in the gay community, but that I really had no choice. They told me to be careful, and we didn't speak of the new disease again—until my own friends and lovers started dying two years later.

Whatever happened during that lunch brought us much closer together. I don't know if my parents would ever come to a wedding, should it ever be possible for me to have one, but they've been with me at a number of memorial services. They're still basically conservative Christians, but despite dogma and theology, both treat me as a son and a fellow Christian. They'll never join PFLAG (Parents and Friends of Lesbians and Gays) or anything, but I don't feel abandoned. When the PFLAG contingent does march down Market Street in the Gay Freedom Day Parade, my eyes always water at the parental support and affection that beam from the faces of others. Yet I always consider that my own parents love and support me in the ways that they can.

During this time Gabe had become my family, my friend, my mother and brother. We had fooled around, of course. Almost all of my friendships started out sexually. But ours was a different sort of romance. We weren't really each other's sexual types, our tastes and preferences tending to be more similar than complementary. We both understood that in the gay community lovers tended to come and go. Both of us yearned for the stability of family based on love and not troubled with romance. And so we made a commitment to live together always, to never leave each other for a career or another man. Lovers were allowed, of course, but they were not to come between us. Gabe was my family man. He helped me enormously as I broke up with Steve and reconnected with my parents. With a few partners we managed to buy a Victorian building and by 1984 lived up and downstairs from each other, like Lucy and Ethel.

My ex-lover, Steve, and I continued to have dinner together at least once a week after I moved out. I still loved him, but I didn't hurt anymore—until 1985 when Steve started having health problems. He was exhausted much of the time, and his gait was changing. He told me he had trouble getting an erection and difficulty with urination. Then he had two small seizures. The doctors did not know what was wrong. He was losing weight, partially, I thought, due to his not having enough energy to prepare meals. But I knew it was a variation on the theme that had already started plaguing our lives.

By late summer 1985 three friends had already died—Mickey, Jesse, Chuck—and Steve was getting worse. His family and friends had been watching him deteriorate for a year, and all of us were frightened. Steve was living alone in Oakland, so we assembled a support group to ensure that he would be safe and cared for, one of thousands of such groups forming across the country. Then he snapped.

It was a typical September morning in San Francisco. I was on my way to work a weekend shift as a nursing supervisor at a local hospital. On the way I stopped in a restaurant near my house and found Steve in the midst of a grand mal seizure. In those days paramedics were not allowed to give antiseizure medications intravenously. By the time the ambulance came and we got to a hospital, Steve had been seizing for almost twenty-five minutes. I don't remember his vital signs, but his blood gases strongly suggested he might need artificial life support.

There was no time to give in to the tide of emotions welling up inside. Now I had to be a nurse. The chief of neurosurgery was called in and wanted to put Steve on a respirator. I explained that he had given me durable power of attorney for his health care and that, as I was responsible for the decision, I needed to understand the rationale before agreeing to it. I explained that I taught nursing and assured the neurosurgeon that I could understand his language and reasoning, but all he would say was, "You mustn't tie the doctor's hands," and "You don't want to second-guess what Steve would want." He concluded our conversation by saying something about my not understanding the difference between life support and a Code Blue (cardiopulmonary resuscitation).

Don't try to second-guess what Steve would want! Isn't that my job? I asked myself. I had known Steve for over eight years. He had been my lover for more than five of those years. For the last twelve months I'd been watching him deteriorate neurologically. In addition, he had asked me to be his durable power of attorney for health care. Who else should try to second-guess what he wanted?

Steve was an attorney. He had written the power of attorney, which excluded the sometimes standard section that says, "If two physicians conclude . . ." When I asked him why, he said that the clause could be construed to give physicians decision-making authority he did not want them to have. Steve hated physicians. His fifty-four-year-old father had had a cardiac history and had died during a hernia repair. Steve and I did not have long discussions about the durable power of attorney, but I remembered several things: "No respirator. No intensive care units. I trust you, Muchkiss [his term of endearment]. You're Supernurse."

However, the physician wouldn't talk to me, and I needed his expertise to help me make this decision. I hadn't worked in critical care for a number of years and was fully aware of my own limitations. So I called Rena, a nurse I had taught with at the vocational nursing school. Then I called Steve's brother in New York. He said he trusted me to make the right decisions and would be on the next flight out.

Rena arrived at the hospital within ten minutes. "Your job is to convince me to put him on the respirator," I told her. Rena did an assessment, consulted with the nurse caring for Steve in the emergency department, and made an impressive argument. When she had finished, we looked at each other and I asked, "Is that it?" She shook her head and hugged me. Both of us knew it was not enough. There was the risk of his giving up and dying because of the insult to the psyche that respirators often bring. And there was his own expressed desire not to ever be on one. It meant I had to be ready to let him die. I did, however, agree to his being placed in the intensive care unit (ICU). What the hell did Steve know about ICUs? I asked myself. He was certainly in no condition to be cared for on a ward. The purpose of a durable power of attorney is to transfer decision-making authority to a trusted person, not to spell out all of the decisions that might need to be made. I had to stand in for Steve, and that meant sending him to ICU. But I'd better be clear about the parameters with both the resident and the charge nurse of the ICU: no heroics—no feeding tubes, no respirator, no code. If Steve was going to make it, he would have to do it without these.

When he woke up a few hours later, he was confused and combative, so the ICU nurses were happy to let one of us stay with him at all times. Three days later he was transferred to a ward with weakness in both legs and some difficulty with his speech. We had a diagnosis: AIDS-related progressive multifocal leukoencephalopathy—a progressive degeneration of the white matter in the brain. Steve's condition was terminal.

Steve was finally discharged, and for the next four months I organized twenty-four-hour care at his home in Oakland. I had become a home-care nurse. As one friend after another fell ill, I remained a home-care nurse—for more than a decade.

For the first month or so Steve was able to get up with help, but he did not move about much in the bed. I wrote a detailed nursing care plan. Turn every two hours. Play music at all times when the television is not on. Get him up for dinner each night. Dinner would be in the dining room with friends. I usually helped feed Steve, although at first he was sometimes able to eat by himself. He had developed a small bedsore in the hospital. It took me two months to heal it. We discovered the wonders of blow-dryers—both for keeping the wound dry and for maintaining general skin care. I wondered why hospitals had not discovered that blow-dryers worked far better than heat lamps or towels. I thought someday I might write an article about it.

We instituted a systematic program to regulate his bowels. Because he was too weak to gulp down eight ounces of fluid with a bulk laxative, we soaked whole psyllium seeds and fed them to him in yogurt or custard. He could not urinate on his own and required frequent catheterization. After several days we resorted to a permanent catheter. Despite some concerns that the sun was bad for AIDS patients, we took Steve out on his patio several times a week. He was a sun worshiper, and retaining some of what was good in his life seemed more important than doing everything possible to prolong it.

The respirator decision seemed like the biggest one we would have to face—until Steve's temperature suddenly spiked up to 105 degrees and he nearly lost consciousness. The likely cause was an infection of the blood that could probably be treated with hospitalization and intravenous antibiotics. I knew that Steve was dying and that his function would never improve. I knew that infections of the blood were one way that nature worked to achieve death. I knew that it was not the worst way of accomplishing the inevitable. However, Steve had never said, "No intravenous antibiotics." Nor should he have been expected to. He designated me to make those decisions, knowing that I was a nurse and would consider what was in his best interest.

What would Steve have decided had he been able to choose? It was important that I not allow my own grief and unwillingness to say goodbye to push us ever further into the world of hospital treatments. Nonetheless, a few more weeks or months like the last few would not be without value. Steve was doing something, I believed. He ate when we fed him. He responded when we came into the room. He was not shutting out the world entirely.

I needed to be certain that Steve was not in physical, psychological, or spiritual pain. So I double-checked my assessment with every person who came to see him. Their responses confirmed my own conclusion. We were suffering, but Steve was really doing okay. He was fighting, holding on—something he said he never wanted to do. But I was responsible to the Steve of today. I had to discern what the Steve of today wanted. I had to act on his behalf. If he was fighting, we would fight. We made two more trips back to the hospital to treat blood infections. I put up a Christmas tree in his bedroom and one in the living room as well.

January came. Steve still ate, but with much less enthusiasm and involvement. He still recognized us some of the time, but the light was off more than it was on. He spent more time in a kind of fugue state—not a vegetable state—but not as good as he had been before Christmas. His closest friends were all saddened at his not dying. I was sad, too, but felt that some preparatory process of a psychological or spiritual nature might be at work. But even that seemed to be disappearing.

I reviewed his care plan. I had decided not to hospitalize Steve should he develop another blood infection. I was prepared to let him go and started to wonder why I was still giving him antibiotics to prevent infections. It was clear that Steve had moved into the last phase; continuing the oral antibiotics as a preventive measure didn't make sense to me anymore. What was my rationale for the antibiotics? It seemed as if I had constructed a little fence to make it more difficult for him to die. He didn't have much energy to spend on dying, and I was going to make him crawl over it, dig under it, or find some other way around my little antibiotic fence. Funny, I didn't question the appropriateness of feeding him, turning him, and caring for him in a myriad of other ways. Our nursing care was probably doing more to keep him alive than the antibiotics were, but how could we do otherwise? As long as he was with us, we would care for him. But the antibiotic fence—was that care, or was it more like intrusive parenting that actually interferes with normal development?

I finally decided to discontinue the oral antibiotics, but Steve's brother, Andrew, disagreed with my decision. To him, stopping the antibiotics was tantamount to pulling the plug. I convened a meeting with Andrew and all of Steve's closest friends. Whereas Andrew was straight and the rest of us were lesbian or gay, we had all been like family for many years. We liked each other. A culture clash was definitely not an issue. Andrew loved his brother more than anyone else in the world, and I respected that love.

Andrew understood the fence analogy but felt that a fence was exactly what was called for. I argued that nature might be more severe, that dying another way might cause a great deal more suffering. Andrew understood but still felt that these were insufficient reasons for discontinuing the antibiotics. As a nurse I needed a rationale for giving a medication, and giving a medication to prevent a condition we had agreed not to treat seemed contradictory. Andrew had agreed with my decision to let Steve go should he get another blood infection. But he argued that he was not a nurse and hence needed no rationale for continuing the preventive antibiotics.

I finally announced that Steve had not asked me to convene a committee to decide what to do. Consensus was desirable but not required. Everyone's concern was important to me. Steve would not have wanted me to disregard his brother's feelings, but he must have known Andrew would find it too difficult to make the ultimate decisions that he had asked me to make.

Andrew was leaving that evening for New York and for some reason desperately wanted to see Steve again before I took him off the antibiotics. We all explained that it was not like pulling the plug, but Andrew was not satisfied. I agreed to one more week on the antibiotics. Andrew would have to fly back the next weekend to see Steve before I discontinued them. After all, I thought, one more week probably wouldn't make that much difference. At the end of that week Steve had another seizure and lapsed into a coma. I never had to enact my decision about his treatment. The whole issue evaporated in an instant and grief filled the vacuum. Andrew arrived Friday night and at 10:00 on Saturday morning, February 1, 1986, Steve died. It was three years to the day since I had moved out.

My parents, brothers, and young nephew came to the memorial service we held in Steve's home. The rabbi from the gay synagogue officiated, and I talked about the similarities between nursing the dying and helping birth babies. Gabe gave the eulogy and read two letters Steve had written, one at age ten to his father in which he accused his brother of misbehaving, the second to the manager of the local supermarket complaining about the service he had received after requesting reimbursement for a rancid chateaubriand. My brother met a colleague of mine at Steve's service. Three years later I was the best man at their wedding. Life had come full circle. Those of us who survived would experience it all over again—death making love more precious; love making death more painful.

Love and Loss: Duckus

The gym where Gabe and I worked out was a virtual menagerie of gay men, and like Adam, Gabe ordered his kingdom by naming the creatures according to their basic traits. Beefers and Blond Boys were easy species to recognize, but Düters were one of his favorites. Düters sat atop two thick thighs and a full round butt and couldn't be more than five feet, nine inches tall. They might have muscled arms, chests, or shoulders, but their distinguishing feature was a visible gravitational force flowing from their trunks to the earth. Düters stood as mirror opposites to Ponies. Düters couldn't fly, but they were very comforting to fire and air types like Gabe and me. But of all the creatures in his kingdom, Ducks were the most difficult to describe.

Gabe said Ducks needed to be seen and experienced. Physically they looked a lot like Düters, but without the gravity. Their skin was watery and usually very smooth. A Duck's lips were full, but had a somewhat peculiar relationship to his nose. "If you put a Duck into the bathtub," Gabe once explained, "he will quack." Ducks were not nearly as numerous as the other species, so it took me a bit longer to recognize them. But eventually I was even able to recognize a subspecies. My lover Martin was a Duck. He wasn't smooth like Ducks normally were. His chest was covered with blond hair, and when Gabe and I considered what it might be like to put him into a bathtub, we weren't sure whether he would quack or bite. So we called him the Biting Duck. He was a dancer turned bodybuilder, buffed from bottom to top. And he made me swoon.

Martin Weber had a lover, and he never noticed me noticing him until after they broke up. We started to banter a bit at the gym. On Memorial Day 1985 the Market Street gym was closed and we found each other at the branch on Hayes Street. I had just finished working out and walked into the locker room. He was seated in the Jacuzzi and silently motioned with his index finger for me to join him. We went to my place. After we had sex, I knew that something wonderful would happen if we could manage to have dinner together. We both canceled our previous plans, went to dinner, and fell in love.

I remember the exact moment. We were eating at the Neon Chicken when he simply said, "I'm a Christian," something not often heard on a date in the Castro. What moved me even more than our shared spiritual beliefs was his simple candor. He was no more like Steve than the sun was like the moon, except that both were beautiful. He worked as a hairdresser and served as a deacon at the Golden Gate Metropolitan Community Church. The Biting Duck proved too difficult a name, and he just didn't seem like a Martin. So Gabe and I called him Duckus.

While Duckus and I were falling in love, Steve was getting sick. Steve's major seizure happened about three months after Duckus and I started seeing each other, and the incident made Duckus decide that both of us needed to take the HIV test that had just become available that year. Not surprisingly, we were both positive.

While I cared for Steve, Gabe actually saw more of Duckus than I did. Duckus never really had me all to himself. I was either caring for Steve or mourning his death. I had planned to spend the anniversary of Steve's death with Sherman, his best friend. But two weeks before that anniversary Duckus's slight flu turned into pneumocystis pneumonia, and he was hospitalized.

My grief would have to wait until my newly scheduled therapy appointments or for a more appropriate time. I couldn't "be there" with Duckus and at the same time give in to the immense feelings of anguish and sadness. For the first week I simply had to help Duckus absorb the shock of the diagnosis, but in general the ways in which I needed to support him were less dramatic than the ways I nursed Steve. The decisions weren't about respirators or no respirator, and Duckus was always fully able to participate in determining his care. Yet there was nursing to do.

In the hospital Duckus was treated with one antibiotic until his blood work forced a change to another one. His breathing was improving, but he got extremely nauseated about an hour after they started infusing the drug. Typically antinausea medication is given thirty minutes prior to infusions, but because Duckus got nauseated about an hour into the treatment, I suggested giving the antinausea drug in the middle of the infusion. That helped. Running the medication in a little faster also helped. These were the sorts of things I was able to figure out by sitting with him hour after hour, day after day.

By February 1 Duckus was doing much better. I had planned to see Sherman and get to the hospital for Duckus's 2:00 P.M. medication, but Duckus called to ask me to come in earlier. An infectious disease specialist was on call for our regular physician, an internist. He asked Duckus how he was doing, and Duckus told him he was nauseous. The doctor offered to discontinue the offending antibiotic and to begin a new course of an experimental drug that Duckus would need to be on

for three more weeks. Duckus was due to complete the regular antibiotic in two or three days, so he wanted me to come in earlier to talk with
him about it.

I didn't think the treatment change made sense. I cared about
Duckus's discomfort with the nausea as much as anyone, but the
change did not seem appropriate. We could wait until Monday when
our regular physician would be back. By Tuesday morning Duckus
would be finished with the original treatment plan.

This on-call doctor and I discussed the matter in Duckus's room.
Finally, more to end the mounting tension than anything else, Duckus
said he would sign papers to begin the experimental medication. I then
did what must have appeared to be very manipulative. I turned to
Duckus, told him he was very tired, told him I wanted to discuss it further, but that I wanted him to make the decision in an unpressured
atmosphere. He assented to this request, and the physician left to chart
that I was interfering with Duckus's care.

With the pressure off, Duckus decided to wait. Once we started on
the experimental medication, our regular physician would have to pre-
tend to support the move, whether he did or didn't. We both wanted
Dr. Wallen to decide if Duckus should have the experimental medication. We'd wait a day and a half. When our own doctor did return, he
was floored that someone had suggested an additional three weeks of
experimental therapy when we had just three days to go with a drug
that was working. Duckus was discharged two days later without needing additional medication.

Even though I had a durable power of attorney for Duckus, I had no
legal authority to intervene because Duckus was fully competent. But
he was also weak. He did not have unlimited energy for informed consent, autonomous decision making, self-advocacy, and discussions with
doctors. Sometimes people just "know" when their friends or loved ones
are acting under duress. This happened twice with Duckus. As he was
being admitted to the hospital for what turned out to be the last time,
he made a point of asking me to bring him home to die. A few days later
when we were told that Duckus was in liver and kidney failure and
would last only a few more days, Duckus said he wouldn't mind staying in the hospital. Everyone heard him, but I didn't buy it. What was
he doing? Was he trying to protect us? I sent everyone out of the room.
After a while I asked Duckus if he was worried about getting up the
forty-five stairs to our flat, and he said he just couldn't do it. When I

explained that I could get him up on a stretcher, he happily agreed to come home.

Back to School

Under ordinary conditions Duckus might have died in the hospital instead of at home. He would certainly have received the experimental medication. Similarly, Steve would have been put on the respirator and there would have been little or no question about the antibiotics. But ordinarily doctors and nurses don't know their patients as well as I knew Steve and Duckus. The long-term, loving relationships I had with them made it possible to care in a personal, rather than in a standard, way.

For better or worse, that was always the way I approached HIV and AIDS—person by person. Research studies and standards of care provide guidelines for clinicians, but often even the best clinicians have to put extra effort into seeing the person behind the disease. This particular disease had grown so large that the people who lived with it might have disappeared altogether had not so many of them resisted the "patient" role. But these newly liberated and often still angry young men were not always easy to understand. I was one of them, and if I couldn't comprehend their issues and concerns, I wondered who would. That was one reason I went back to school—to develop a richer and more sensitive understanding of my friends who were also coping with HIV.

Another reason for my going back to school was that Samuel Merritt College started encouraging its faculty to earn their doctoral degrees. I knew I might well be dead in the five years or so it would take me to finish a Ph.D., but what if I put my career on hold and then stayed healthy? What would I say to myself—oh, I might have been a good professor, but I thought I was going to die? The idea of being depressed after living five or ten years longer than my friends and lovers seemed ridiculous. It was a perfect time. None of the people I loved was sick. Duckus died in November 1987, and by September 1988 I was back in school.

Whenever I happen to die, I am convinced that a heavenly committee will review the demographic summary of my earthly incarnation: gay man, nurse, teacher, student; lived in San Francisco during the AIDS epidemic. So in addition to satisfying the tenure requirements of my employer, I had to satisfy my friends on the other side. My research focus would have to be HIV, and my heavenly committee would take no bullshit. They would not be impressed with big federal grants.

Although I knew I wasn't expected to find the cure for AIDS, research-ing hypotheses from the social sciences such as "People are less likely to follow through with decisions about safer sex when they are drunk" would surely get me a ticket to the most tedious part of hell.

Friends with HIV were constantly asking for my opinions, and I felt obligated to offer the most intellectually defensible and individually rel-evant advice possible. To do this, I had to discover how population-based science intersected with the artful expression of life that varied so much from person to person. I had to take the sidewalk discussions in our community more seriously. I had to pay closer attention to what HIV meant in individual lives.

My dissertation work was organized around the metaphors of war and religion. During the years I spent rewriting and reevaluating the central meanings in my stories, I dropped some of my earlier emphasis on these metaphors. Nonetheless, they merit brief mention here.

War is the most overt metaphor in modern medicine, and it is employed in response to all diseases. But modern medicine isn't the only discipline guided by this metaphor. The metaphor of war has sig-nified our response to an increasing number of medical and social prob-lems. Lyndon Johnson started a war on poverty. Richard Nixon declared war on cancer. Retired generals wage a war on drugs. Emmanuel Dreuilhe wrote a moving book about a war against AIDS fought on the battleground of his own body.[3] Social liberals admonished us to "fight AIDS, not people with AIDS."

But there were pacifists, even in this war. My friend Jason often spoke of "making peace" with the virus. Others accepted the war metaphor but questioned strategy, particularly our overinvestment and conse-quent overreliance on the offensive weapons of medical intervention. To these more holistically minded folk, our preoccupation with advanced weaponry diverted attention from defensive concerns—the health, well-being, and combat readiness of our immune systems; the availability of fresh food and water; and related psychological and envi-ronmental conditions.

Whereas biomedicine unabashedly took up the metaphor of war, the ways in which it took up the metaphor of religion were less obvious. For decades scholars from a variety of disciplines have discussed the paral-lels between Western biomedicine and state religions and several have noted that the health care system has taken over many responsibilities that once adhered to the church. Today the modern hospital supervises our births, our suffering, and our deaths. But most importantly, the bio-medical industry supervises the production of truth through officially sanctioned research. Like the Catholic Church of the Middle Ages, the biomedical industry has become a monolithic power that structures not only what we understand as "knowledge," but also the way we feel about and understand ourselves in relation to sickness, suffering, and death.

Yet there are big differences between modern medicine and the modern church. In the Western world it is possible to reject modern religion. But it is as impossible to walk away from modern medicine as it was to walk away from the church of the Middle Ages. The sacrament of health care can be withheld, as it frequently is in the United States, where more than 40 million people still live without health insurance, but the importance of health care cannot be denied. Nonetheless, heathens and heretics have never been completely extinguished.

I came to appreciate that being a nurse is somewhat like being a nun. Nuns are told what to profess by a religious hierarchy, whereas nurses obtain their doctrine from an industrial or academic one. But the truths perpetuated by our religions and sciences are far more orderly than the real world in which people live—worlds of crisis, chaos, and ambiguity. Nuns and nurses tend to live closer to the people than do their more powerful counterparts. Consequently, both nuns and nurses often wind up mediating relationships between their neighbors and the larger powers that govern twentieth-century life.

Today many nurses act as apologists or even evangelists for the medical status quo. Many nurses (especially those in academic positions) demonstrate a deep reverence toward the modern systems charged with developing scientific knowledge. They are contemptuous toward the "n of one," the anecdote, the individual patient. But other nurses revere the sanctity of specific human lives more than they do statistical data based on populations and aggregates. My own challenge was to remain simultaneously respectful and skeptical of both positions. The following ten stories tell what I learned and to what degree I met that challenge.

| 3 |

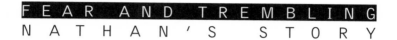

FEAR AND TREMBLING
NATHAN'S STORY

The "Christmas Fairies" were conceived at the Muscle System Gym in 1987 just after Duckus died. His mother requested that an old hymn— "I come to the gar-den a-lone; while the dew is still on the ro-ses"—be sung at his memorial service. I loved the hymn, but it seemed too maudlin, too self-indulgent, for Duckus. My solution was to get eight guys together to sing it barbershop style, in four-part male harmony. Notwithstanding the nature of our debut, the eight of us had such a good time that we decided to have a few more rehearsals and go Christmas caroling together.

The group grew to about fifteen. Those who couldn't read music sang the melody. On Fridays and Sundays we sang at a hospital or two and then hit the bars, crashed parties, or marched down Castro Street spreading cheer and drinking hot brandies. Nathan, a Muscle System regular with a big bass voice, joined us in 1988. A few weeks after Christmas we bumped into each other at the gym. He was still glowing from the caroling experience and in the course of a quick conversation between sets mentioned he'd just started AZT.

Ordinarily we would have continued the conversation on the corner before walking to our respective cars. I'd had so many conversations, important conversations, like this with guys from the gym. This time I mentioned my study, and Nathan agreed to talk with me on tape. We met at his house the next day.

A recent transplant from Washington, D.C., Nathan was in the middle of his psychiatric residency. We settled into the big sofa next to the piano. I flipped on the recorder and got quickly to the point: "What I basically want to get is your story. How has HIV affected your life?"

"Wow! Big question. In a hundred words or less. Well, it was about 1981. I was in my second year of medical school and wasn't feeling very good. I had just had hepatitis B and was having a hard time snapping back from it. About two months later I developed swollen lymph nodes. I was the one who was first concerned about AIDS. The doctor hadn't heard about it yet. He told me not to worry—it was such a rare thing. But it was on my mind from that point forward. It never left. I felt lousy during most of that year—like having mono. It was hard for me to concentrate on my studies, so I took some time off from medical school.

"About a year later I was living in New York, and in New York people were talking about AIDS. There wasn't much in the *New York Times*, but people were talking everywhere, handing out pamphlets on the streets, and getting hysterical. I just soaked up the AIDS hysteria and got depressed. I was sure I had it—whatever it was—and thought it was probably a virus.

"So I went to see an AIDS specialist, and she did skin testing. This is great. Good story. I'd already finished two years of medical school, so I knew what skin testing meant. She kept shaking her head. The message I got from her was, 'You are typical; you are doomed.' I was supposed to come back and have the results read, but I didn't have any reaction to the skin tests, and rather than realizing that that was a bad sign, I just totally blocked it out. I was in total denial. I've never had a case of denial that extreme in my life. I canceled my appointment and the nurse told me I had to come in and have my skin test read. And I just said, 'Don't worry. I'm fine. I'm fine.'"

"Did you know what having no reaction to the skin tests meant?"

"Let's put it this way: I may not have known what it really meant, but it would have taken about thirty seconds to figure it out."

"Did we know we were dealing with an immune problem at that point?"

"Yes. We definitely did. It's real elementary. Then I forgot I had ever done the test until a whole year later. It terrified me because it meant I had no immune system. Then one day after I was back in medical school, I was doing skin testing on somebody. All of a sudden I remembered my own skin test, and the result, and I was horrified. But during the year I was off from medical school, I started feeling great. I moved to Puerto Rico and was just lying on the beach and sleeping and playing and having a great time. And I started feeling much, much better, like myself again. I guess for that whole period of time—it's hard to remember back—I lived in fear. But there was a fair amount of denial. There were so few people who had died from this thing that I was sure I wouldn't be one of them. I used to make an analogy with hepatitis B—I got sick initially, developed antibodies, and now am fine. I thought the people who died of AIDS were probably the ones who never formed antibodies, like the chronic hepatitis B carriers. So I thought I was probably fine and that nothing more would happen. That was my theory, and it allowed me to keep going and not get totally paranoid.

"In December 1984 on a routine physical my platelets came back at 60,000, normal being close to 150,000. So that really flipped me out. The doctor didn't really know what to make of it until a week later when the *New England Journal of Medicine* came out with an article about HIV-related thrombocytopenia [low platelets]. So we figured it was that. So once again I had never been tested, but there was no doubt in my mind."

"The test wasn't even available yet, was it?" I asked.

"That's right. When did they have the test?"

"Around 1985."

"That was when I moved to San Francisco, in May of 1985. And that was when I started having safe sex. Up until that time people in D.C. weren't having safe sex. When I came here, people were. So I just did what everybody else was doing. When I look back, I can't believe that D.C. was so far behind."

"You went to med school in D.C.?"

"Right. After I moved here, I would alternate between being depressed, freaking out, being scared, and being in denial. I really couldn't escape it here. People were sick all around, and the *B.A.R.* [a weekly gay newspaper] with their obituaries every week! So there were periods where I felt hopeless about it and periods where I felt okay about it. I'd just sort of fluctuate back and forth.

"A year and a half later, in the spring of '86, I went to get tested. I didn't really want to do it, though. I was terrified of the social ramifications. If I didn't know my antibody status, then I could always tell people, 'Well, I don't know.' But if I was positive, I felt I would be obligated to tell people, and I was afraid nobody would want to be with me. So as long as I didn't know, it was easy, but as soon as I knew, I'd have a certain responsibility that I didn't want to have. Even though I knew I was positive anyway, I could always say I hadn't been tested. So I got the test and then freaked out, changed my mind, and never went to find out the results."

▼ ▼ ▼

Not only did Nathan face the possibility of a terminal illness; he also faced being rejected or radically redefined by his own people. A new set of symbols, standards, behaviors, and judgments was reshaping sexuality in San Francisco and had already changed Nathan's sexual practices. His comment about having safe sex in San Francisco but not in D.C. demonstrates the power of community structures and norms on individual sexual practices. Nathan tended to do "what everybody else was doing," in both cities. The new medical labels were constructing new social identities. Once Nathan accepted one of those medical labels, he knew there would be no turning back. New "responsibilities" would follow him into the bedroom, into his intimate relationships. Initially, all these possibilities proved to be overwhelming. But in San Francisco even partial denial was much more difficult to sustain.

▼ ▼ ▼

"Then in the spring of '87 I went for a routine physical and my white count came back at 3.9 [low]. And my doctor said, 'You have to get tested because this is an indication that something might be wrong, and there is really no excuse not to get tested at this point.' So I agreed to go ahead and finally get tested. I felt I really had to face it and was fully prepared for a positive result. What I wasn't fully prepared to find out was that my T cells were only 226. So what happened actually was that I got the results of the T cells before I got the results of the HIV test.

"I'll never forget it. It was Friday evening at 7:00. I was just about to go out and the phone rang; it was my doctor and he said, 'I have the results of your test.' And my knees just went weak and I started shaking all over. He said, 'The first one is the T cells. Are you sitting down?' Oh God, what an asshole. I was really pissed. I thought he was joking. Like why? It was such a stupid thing to say."

"Lots of doctors never learn how to talk to people."

"I think he learned something because I gave him shit. He said, 'Are you sitting down?' And I said, 'Yeah, go ahead, what?—what!' My knees were weak and I was getting shaky and my heart was racing and he said, '226.' I went totally—I've never reacted like that to any situation in my life—I went completely into panic. I was on the floor. I could barely speak. I was hyperventilating. Then after I gathered my wits about me, I yelled at him and told him it was really a stupid thing to do. I said, 'How could you call me at home and tell me something like this?' And he said, 'Are you okay?' I said, 'I'm fine; I'm fine. I just need to get off the phone.' He was all freaked out and didn't want to let me off the phone and said, 'Are you sure you are going to be okay?' I said I was fine, I just needed to get off this damn phone, and I slammed the phone down and popped a Xanax. I laid down on the bed and immediately called my best friend in D.C. I was shaking so much that the telephone was rattling against my ear. I could barely hold it still to talk. I remember when the Xanax finally took effect because my hand finally stopped shaking.

"What freaked me out so much was that I wasn't familiar with the numbers and I really didn't know what they meant. I had just learned about what the ranges were. I had heard that 200–400 was ARC. So immediately in my mind I had ARC. Anything under 200 meant you were vulnerable to opportunistic infections. I didn't know anything about how T cells could stay in the same place for a long time. Actually, I didn't know anything. Even being a doctor, I didn't know anything. So what I thought that meant was that any day I would come down with AIDS. It was like, 'Sorry I have to tell you this, but you only have a year to live.'

"None of the doctors knew what they meant either. It was through my own experience, through what I learned from other people, through watching my own numbers. But it wasn't from having learned it from a textbook or from an article because even now nobody really knows."

▼▼▼

As a nurse I didn't always understand the numbers either. Because we hadn't been doing T-cell counts before, there was no history, no context in which to interpret them. We digressed to discuss how another laboratory value was being constructed. Ratios were out; percents were in.[1] Of course, we didn't really know what the "percents" meant either, but people with relatively high CD4 cells who got opportunistic infections tended to have a lower percentage of CD4 cells to total lymphocytes. Some physicians suggested that people take medication to prevent pneumocystis pneumonia when the percent of CD4s to total lymphocytes dropped below 20. After arguing over a few details the way doctors and nurses sometimes do, we returned to Nathan's story.

▼ ▼ ▼

"Probably the most biological, classical, major depression of my life followed that phone call. It was the only time in my life that I really couldn't eat. I had this lump in my throat. It was hard to swallow. I lost five pounds. I could barely get out of bed. I did, but barely. I felt completely hopeless. I was more stunned than weepy. I was mostly numbed. I wasn't really crying a lot, after the first day. I was just in shock, for seven days.

"Then I had my T cells rechecked, and they were 315 a week later. So I learned my first lesson about T cells from that. They could vary 100 points. It didn't really mean anything necessarily."

▼ ▼ ▼

Nathan's comment that "it didn't really mean anything necessarily" is often used by both doctors and patients, but its meaning is often ambiguous. The phrase was repeated several times by the men in my study and rarely meant the same thing twice. When Nathan said, "It didn't really mean anything necessarily," he meant that he wasn't necessarily going to get sick and die within the year.

Though a medical student, Nathan's interpretation of his own skin test was not scientific but symbolic. The negative skin test indicated not a compromised immune system but no immune system. Even physicians occasionally interpret laboratory tests within personal, rather than rational, frameworks. In fact, nobody understands laboratory tests in perfectly rational and abstract terms all of the time. Nor should we. Despite our culture's having come to idolize the rational over the past three hundred years, much of life is lived outside neat rational abstractions in the rather messy world of personal and social meanings and concerns. This is not to say that all personal meanings should be accepted without argument, but rather that in health care personal and social meanings and rational constructs must meet on some sort of common ground. Nathan seemed to find that common ground, often by moving back and forth between his feelings and his science. Having no immune system whatsoever was way too dangerous to Nathan's sense of self, so he "forgot" that he had taken the test for a whole year, perhaps the most rational response possible.

In our conversation Nathan characterized his response as "total denial." He didn't say whether this denial was a healthy or pathological defense mechanism, but it was not all-encompassing. He did not continue as if everything were normal; he took a year off from medical school. In addition, he needed more than a vague sense of hope. He needed a specific understanding that was hopeful for him, so he constructed an analogy between HIV and hepatitis B that indicated he would not be among those who were dying.

Unlike the skin test results, which had to be repressed, Nathan's low platelet and low white blood cell counts represented no immediate danger or threat. Those tests simply supported his presumption that he had "whatever it was." Nathan was able to accept the *New England Journal of Medicine's* explanation of HIV-related thrombocytopenia as the reason for his low platelet count, but in 1986 he could not bring himself to have his supposition confirmed. He got tested, panicked, and could not go back for the results. In 1987 when he took the HIV test again, the emotional weight—the freak-out factor of confirming what he already "knew"—was eclipsed by news of a new medical measurement, the CD4 count. His entire story about getting his "test result" is focused on the CD4 count, not the antibody test.

"Even being a doctor," Nathan didn't "know anything." But "in his mind" there were meanings, interpretations, reactions. Nathan did not rationally choose the meanings he assigned to these numbers. He interpreted them—reacted to them—in the context in which they were given—"Are you sitting down?" We had the medical technology to measure CD4 counts in 1987, but not the experience necessary to make much sense of them. Neither his medical education nor his psychiatric residency did much to reduce Nathan's terror or the symbolic interpretations that grew out of it. So he turned to "alternative things."

▼ ▼ ▼

"I decided to start researching everything I could possibly do for myself. AZT wasn't a possibility at that time. It was still just experimental.

There were really no treatments at that point. So I just went completely into all the alternative things. I came across one of those newsletters, *Healing AIDS Naturally*. I've always been somewhat holistically minded. So within a week after being in a major depression I was out there doing—let me think—there is a whole list. First I started doing complete vitamin therapy," he said, laughing, "like several hundred dollars on vitamins. I got this list and I bought every single one on the list. I started doing acupuncture, Chinese herbs. I started jogging regularly, meditating, visualization.

"Six months previously I had started reading *A Course in Miracles*, which is the first spiritual work that ever touched me in any way. It had been collecting dust in a corner, so I pulled that out again. I started reading things like Louise Hay,[2] Dr. Bernie Siegel, a lot of inspirational things about mind over body. I joined a support group at the Center for Attitudinal Healing, which I attended for fifteen months." He started laughing again. "That was it. Then I took six months off from my residency while I was instituting all of these things. I came out to my supervisor and training director. I told them what was going on, and they were very supportive. So I was given the time off with pay, which was really nice."

"Jesus! You did it all. What was that like?"

"It was empowering. It gave me the feeling that I could have control over this, particularly when I read things from Louise Hay and Bernie Siegel. I also attended seminars and whatnot. I got it into my mind that I'm not going to be a victim of this. I can take charge. I can have control over this. And my theory at the time—it's changed significantly since then—was that if I don't want to die, I'm not going to die. I can will this thing into submission," he laughed. "And I needed to feel that at the time. Everything I was doing for it—the meditation, the vitamins, the herbs—made me feel like this was my way of controlling it. As long as I was doing those things, this thing was not going to get me. I felt real positive about that.

"Throughout the first year I gradually started dropping all the things I had started. I didn't feel like going for acupuncture anymore. The herbs were a pain in the ass—boiling that shit every morning, and the smell was horrible. Not to mention the expense! The herbs and acupuncture cost about $60 or something. And the vitamins were expensive, too. I stuck with the herbs about six weeks. The vitamins even less time. I was taking everything!" he laughed. "All those trace minerals and enzymes; all this shit. Then I started doing AL-721.[3] I did that for an entire year. The only thing it probably did was put weight on me. I finally boiled it down to a multivitamin, multimineral, E and C. So that's what I've been taking since then.

"But again these things were important because they gave me confidence psychologically. I wasn't just sitting there doing nothing. As time went on, I realized I'm still alive and not getting sick. But I needed to do all those things before to give me a sense of power. When I regained confidence that I wasn't ready to drop dead, I was able to stop doing a lot of those things.

"Over the next two years [1987–1989] I alternated between feeling like I had control over it and being in total denial. Sometimes I felt spiritually tuned in—meditating, studying *A Course in Miracles*, and thinking as long as I was leading this kind of very aware life, where I was open and loving and not suppressing a lot of junk, I'd be okay—that was the control phase. There'd be another phase when I was in denial about everything, when I just didn't think about HIV at all, when it became nonexistent.

"I realized, of course, that there was something to worry about, but emotionally I just wasn't thinking about it. I just went about my daily business, going to work, coming home, cooking dinner, and not really thinking about being HIV positive. I would plan for the future and what I was going to do ten years from now—well not ten years. But I would think about next year and the year after that and finishing my residency and what I wanted to do—with no regard to being HIV positive.

"That's what I mean when I say denial. Sometimes I thought I had control over it. But sometimes I was just plugged up, cut off, just going through the motions of life and not thinking about things very much. In some ways it was a grayish, depressed time when I'd do nothing at all. And that would scare me. I would think, I'm not doing anything to help myself right now. I'm not exercising. I'm smoking cigarettes. I'm not doing any kind of treatments. So I'd get scared and think, you've got to do something here. At other times I'd go to my support group. I always liked to have at least one thing. I stopped the support group after about a year.

"As an elective, half-time, I formed a mental health clinic for HIV/AIDS at the VA hospital. Interesting things came up for me there. I had very little empathy for people who came in with a victim consciousness. There were people who came in with ARC who wanted to go onto disability, who were drinking and partying, and it used to piss me off. The hard thing was that I was seeing myself as a victim and it was real hard to see others who were so obvious with it. This was a big issue in my supervision.[4] And I wasn't much better with the ones who had just received their test results. I got so tired of the new people freaked out and saying, 'Oh my God, I'm HIV positive.' I thought, God, I don't want to hear this shit. I was tired of helping people get through the initial parts. I wanted to move on. I didn't want to keep going over and over it. It just seemed like enough was enough. So I quit.

"Then I joined a group for HIV-positive male psychotherapists," he said, laughing. "It was just once a month, and I thought, this will be really great. These people will really be able to process things. I was really looking forward to it. I went once or twice, and then I started building some incredible resistance to going. I realized I didn't want to go to that either, so I quit. I didn't want to sit around talking about it anymore. I just wanted to live. I was so tired of talking about it."

"So what finally convinced you to take AZT?"

"I had a very rigid, pushy, by-the-book internist who said, 'You just have to do this.' But the same day I was told I needed to be on AZT, I was told I needed to go on pentamidine and that I should fill out a durable power of attorney.[5] So I really flipped out. When he gave me the forms for the durable power of attorney, I felt like I was getting a death warrant to sign, whereas a friend of mine immediately filled them out because he said it made him feel much better."

"It gives some people a sense of control."

"Yeah, but that was the same day my ANC [absolute neutrophil count] was 800.[6] My doctor believes in full-strength AZT, and now he thinks, because of the ANC, that I'm in too terrible a state to be on full-strength AZT! I'm now tied to a schedule of getting my arm stuck every two weeks. I have an M.D. visit every two weeks and a once-a-month pentamidine appointment. So now I'll never be able to stop thinking about AIDS. I can never go back. It is just like it was getting tested. I could never go back to saying that I didn't know. These treatments are for life, or until something better comes along, or until I die. And that is real depressing for me.

"But you know what's weird? The guys in the breathing room were so nice to me that I felt bad about it. I was on the other side of the AIDS caregiver role, and it made me feel like a patient. I was in a position that I needed to be nurtured. Later eight guys came into the room, and some of them were very ill. And suddenly I found myself among the ranks of the ill. I knew that it would just be a matter of time and that I would get used to it, and I have. The only thing that still bums me out are the side effects of the AZT."

"What does the AZT mean to you now? Does it mean that you're sick?"

"I used to have a need to say that I'm healthy. Agreeing to take the AZT has brought me to the place of acknowledging that I have a life-threatening condition and that that is okay. There is more of a feeling of acceptance. I'm not fighting against it anymore. I'm not giving up either. But I'm not fighting against my denial. AZT is a symbol of letting go of denial.

"All along I've denied that I've had symptoms, but it's not really true. I really feel like I'm ten years ahead in the aging process. I cannot imagine staying out all night anymore, and I should still be able to do that at thirty-two, and that was going on even before the AZT. I have to get to bed at nine or ten o'clock. One of my biggest fears is dementia. I feel that I have less of a buffer zone in terms of my capacity to insult my brain with substances. The slightest thing will throw off my thinking. For example, when I went on the cruise last April, I let myself go nuts. I drank, did a few drugs, stayed up late. It took me two weeks to recover. My body was okay, but my brain felt sluggish. Whenever I don't get enough sleep, if I have any alcohol, I worry because my brain is not as sharp. This is a continual fear for me—that I might get demented or psychotic."

Not everyone I was to interview experienced conflict over whether they were doing enough to take care of themselves. Nathan vacillated between doing everything (herbs, acupuncture, vitamins, etc.) and doing nothing. Doing nothing darkened the "grayish depression" for a while until he found another way to take care of himself. When that got tiring, he stopped it. Though Nathan is a psychiatrist, even talk got boring, and eventually he stopped that, too.

Three years after our interview, in 1993, Nathan decided he really had been experiencing the differences that come with age as opposed to AIDS. He was not the only one asking the question. Many, many gay men with asymptomatic HIV infection continue to wonder whether their decreased energy is related to AIDS or age. Our friend Kyle used to ask rhetorically, "Is it the Big A or the little a?"

After 1987 AZT was probably the common strategy that people with HIV used to ward off the "Big A," even though it often seemed to accelerate the "little a." But when Nathan started taking AZT, it wasn't because he found his doctor's arguments reasonable or convincing. It wasn't really because he was convinced that it would help. Unlike some of the men whose stories follow, Nathan never said AZT gave him hope. No. Nathan began AZT for two reasons. First, an older, more dominant gay physician was able to push his opinion onto a younger, more vulnerable gay physician. Nathan never really believed in AZT, but he complied with his doctor's recommendation. Second, Nathan needed to let go of some "denial," and AZT would serve to accomplish that for him.

"A few weeks ago you mentioned that you were afraid AZT was a poison," I continued.

"I'm still worried about that. In two and a half years my T cells have stayed relatively constant. My body may have its own wisdom, and the AZT may fuck it up. I was feeling fine without it, and it angers me that now I feel shitty. I really don't have a choice. I feel that I've given the AZT some of my power. If I stopped taking the AZT now, I would feel very vulnerable. So I feel kind of angry and trapped. It makes me feel lousy, but I can't stop. Now, that might not be true. I might stop taking it if I really felt bad month after month."

In fact, Nathan did start feeling bad in a few months and told his doctor he would rather die than take the full dose of AZT. Nathan called me later that day to tell me how "pissed off" his doctor was.

"He was so pissed off that he dictated his notes right in front of me. He turned on the Dictaphone and said, 'Patient refuses to take 500 mg as recommended. Will only take 300 mg even though I told him there is no evidence that 300 mg'. . . blah, blah, blah—as if life waits for evidence. You know, I never thought the AZT did much at all. There never was a bump in my T cells."

▼ ▼ ▼

A couple of years later Nathan had two T-cell counts in a row that were below 200 and he told me, "I got horribly depressed. I thought this is it. It's inevitable. There're two of them now." He started Prozac and his T cells went back to above 200. On the advice of his new physician, Nathan stopped the AZT. He tried two new antivirals. DDC gave him canker sores, and ddI gave him diarrhea. Two months later his T cells went up a bit more. For the next few years Nathan stayed away from antivirals altogether.

Like the HIV test, like the low CD4 count, the pervasive metaphoric power that AZT once had for Nathan eventually crumbled. Eventually, a CD4 count around 200 would no longer mean Nathan was at death's door. Yet the metaphoric power associated with HIV was not confined to personal interpretations, scientific understandings, or the doctor-patient relationship. HIV was also being redefined at the dinner table, in the bedroom, and in casual conversation. Nathan's story about telling his family, people at work, and the guys at the gym reflects his holistic orientation, his hopefulness, and his fears.

▼▼▼

"About three weeks into this whole thing I flew home to visit my family in D.C. It was an emergency sort of thing. I've always been very close to my parents. I needed to tell them, and I didn't want to tell them by phone, but they got all alarmed anyway when they knew I was coming home. I walked in the door and my mother said, 'What is the matter? This is not like you. Why did you come home just like this?' And I said, 'I'm fine, I'm fine, I'm fine.' I didn't want to tell them before dinner because I didn't want to ruin dinner. So we sat down to dinner—and I sat there, still emotional and in shock about the whole thing. I was dreading that moment when dinner ended. Finally my mother looked at me and said, 'Why did you come home?'

"You know, I learned something from the beginning. When I was very upset about it, then anyone I told would get upset about it. Now when I tell people I'm HIV positive, they just go, 'Oh'—and it's no big deal. But at the time we all started crying. So it was that kind of a scene. They were very supportive, and my father and mother and I sat on the couch and huddled together and cried. It was actually a very wonderful supportive moment that I will never forget.

"I was worried that my mother would be too dramatic and hysterical. In fact, both of them struck a really nice balance between being supportive and yet not being in denial—but not being overly dramatic either. I had my Louise Hay tape with me. It was a videotape of the group she had done in L.A. Within an hour after I told them, I popped this video in the VCR and told them, 'See, I don't have to die from this. Listen to these people. I don't want you to feel hopeless about this thing because I'm going to be fine.' They really appreciated that video. My father especially really just loved it, thought it was wonderful stuff. From then on I started educating them. I gave them *Love, Medicine, and Miracles* [by Bernie Siegel]. But there was a big concern about telling my mother because I had always been her support and I didn't want to be her support through this. I wanted her to be my support.

"I found the process of telling people I was HIV positive was sort of like coming out. It was like that all over again—wondering who I could trust enough to say it to—worrying about the rejection, what people would think and whatnot. Interestingly, I was more comfortable telling people at work. I told my whole residency group. I was really afraid that the guys at the gym would somehow all ostracize me. I was afraid no one would want to go out with me. No one would want to sleep with me. No one would want to be my lover. That kind of stuff. So I was actually more afraid for people to know in the gay community."

"Some of us don't give a rat's ass," I replied, "but you're certainly not alone. I've been real surprised at who feels that way. Some people don't mind anyone knowing that they're HIV positive for years, but then when their T cells drop, they don't want anyone to know."

"Exactly. Right. I've felt that way, too. Of course, I was both at the same time. I was HIV positive, and I had low T cells. If I ever did tell anyone I was HIV positive, I just hoped they didn't ask me what my T cells were! Who would want to get involved with somebody who is on the brink of AIDS? T cells in the 200s? People are going to be reading me as being on the brink of being sick. Who'd want to form a relationship with someone about to get sick? It's fine to say, 'I'm HIV positive and my T cells are at 1,200, so I've got enough mileage, or I'm never going to get sick.' But when they're that low, people think that you're going to get sick soon."

▼ ▼ ▼

When Nathan first heard that his T cells were low, he thought the same thing. The medical community had just started saying that a CD4 count of 200 meant ARC, and to Nathan that meant having a year or so to live.

We didn't really talk about death in our first interview, but the subject came up a few years later. Without ever turning into a full-fledged New Age convert, Nathan investigated a number of spiritual ideas and practices. He mentioned a conference he had just attended where someone spoke of two Indian gurus who had recently died of cancer.

"Perhaps part of our soul healing is to experience a death," Nathan told me.

"No shit," I thought silently.

"These two gurus dying of cancer really helped me let go of some of the control."

Death terrified Nathan, in part because it made no metaphysical or spiritual sense to him. The death of two gurus opened up the possibility that death might have some purpose—that it might be something other than a sign of failure. Being relieved of his responsibility to control his own mortality was comforting for Nathan. Yet the death of his father took him much further. His father's death not only shattered his fledgling sense of control; it also obliterated the centrality of Nathan's own personal drama.

▼▼▼

"My father was diagnosed with cancer and given six months to live. After that my own health issues were put aside. My father's illness really became the most important thing. My mother and I spent the next year taking care of him. Dad fought with it all. We even went to Tijuana for Laetrile therapy, and the tumors actually shrank for a while, and he felt real good and everyone went, 'Oh, this is what a positive attitude can do.' But then Dad got sick and died. I did the nursing with my mother for the last two weeks.

"For the next few months I was kind of numbed out. I didn't care much what happened. I didn't do any spiritual work for almost two years after Dad died. I felt pretty jaded much of the time. On top of that one of my very best friends from D.C. had a long, lingering death—horrible. He was one of those people I thought would never progress to AIDS. His death chipped away more of the denial.

"I no longer live in fear, but I don't ignore HIV either. It's just kind of there. I plan for the future now. I'm buying a house, but I no longer feel omnipotent. I no longer have that 'I won't die 'cause I'm me' attitude."

▼▼▼

Nathan's father mounted a valiant struggle, employed Eastern and Western therapies, summoned vast stores of personal fortitude and inner strength, and died. Through this death and the death of his best friend, Nathan gained perspective and a greater sense of connectedness. Although Nathan got "numbed out" with grief, he lost some of his personal terror and sense of isolation. When death became less terrifying, the denial and control strategies he had used to manage it receded. Despite the uncertainty that comes from living with HIV, Nathan looked to the future with as much pragmatism as possible. He had done this before. During our initial interview in 1989 Nathan talked about his decision to finish his residency.

▼▼▼

"I seriously considered dropping out of the residency. I worked ten years toward the goal of being a psychiatrist and thought, if I'm going to die in the next couple of years, why the fuck do I want to kill myself for two more years of residency, only to get sick and not be able to use this stuff? I strongly considered dropping out. I really was tortured by that for a while, until finally I decided to proceed. I started to realize I had no way of predicting the course of this thing, and if two years from then I was still fine and sitting there with ten years of wasted education, I'd be really pissed."

We both laughed, knowing we understood each other and the irony of the situation perfectly. "Of course, we know how that ended," he said. "I actually finished. Thank God I did."

▼▼▼

By 1993 Nathan was off antivirals and life was feeling a bit more normal again. He worked out, looked great, and generally felt pretty good. Over time he found himself working a fifty-hour week again. He also found himself smoking more, drinking more, and playing harder. Nathan's world was full of sorrow, but it was also replete with people, products, and pleasures that he found supportive. Cigarettes helped him engage with the nerve-wracking aspects of his life. Xanax helped calm his nerves. When he needed more energy, testosterone provided it, both during sex and at the gym. When he had too much energy, sleeping pills were there to soak up the excess. Whereas his life was certainly full of difficult challenges, it was also full of pleasure and possibility. In short, as Nathan reengaged with his world, that world helped Nathan to manage, helped him to live.

With the advent of the protease inhibitors in 1996, Nathan decided to try the HIV cocktail. His T cells were still around 200, and his viral load was only 20,000. I made a weak case for waiting, but I knew that he had made up his mind. By then I had known Nathan for more than eight years and was convinced that he knew how to take care of himself. He had stopped smoking and retired from work. He knew how to manage his stress and balance his pleasures and disciplines. As long as drugs didn't make him sick, Nathan would embrace and find hope in them.

In 1998 Nathan is still on the cocktail and his viral load remains undetectable. His T cells are still around 200–300. His only side effect is a sky-high cholesterol, and he is monitoring that. In addition to testosterone, he now does anabolic steroids. He works out like a fiend and looks like a doll (a muscle doll). He's taking courses in the humanities, practicing yoga, meditating, playing the piano, singing Christmas carols, and thinking about going back to work.

This story started in 1981.

| 4 |

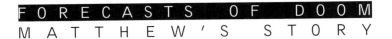

FORECASTS OF DOOM
MATTHEW'S STORY

There was only one reason for a San Francisco homosexual to be on Fourth Street in the middle of the day. Sandwiched between a gas station and a cheap motel, the clap clinic was a venerated San Francisco institution. The first few minutes were always the most awkward. It wasn't standing before the massive desk or facing the dozen or more subaltern officials and clerks who moved behind it. Most of these were occupied with incomprehensible duties, and only one or two attended to the line. No, it was standing with your back to the one or two hundred patients in the seats behind you. These were the people you might know—or might want to know.

To show I was neither intimidated nor repentant, I always wore Levi's and a black leather jacket, but not a trashy shirt. And yet it was all quite awkward. How do you cruise at the clap clinic? And how do you not cruise when you're in a room full of gay men who have nothing else to do? That, together with the fact that the whole flock was "grounded," made the whole thing weird and depressing.

As numbers were called, we watched each other get up and walk to one of the tiny cubicles that lined the room. Between each call, we retook our seats with the rest of the mostly male group. I couldn't tell you what percentage might have been straight because I saw only the gay men. There weren't many prostitutes, though, of either sex. They had long ago learned how to avoid such trouble or else got their care from the privates.

The first call was to an office on the right wall. The social worker had your record—an eight-and-a-half-by-five-and-a-half-inch card with room for about thirty visits. When that filled up, the social worker stapled on a second. I knew a couple of guys who had three. The second call was usually to the physician. Their offices were in a hallway to the left of the main desk in the front. The rectal swab wasn't bad, but the wire they stuck into the penis could really smart. It helped to have a healthy drip so that they wouldn't be as tempted to go probing. The third call was to the nurse who administered injections or gave pills, depending on the protocol. Her quarters were on the left wall, in the rear of the room. Even if you got shots, you usually had to take some pills as well. The water fountain was in the middle of the wall on the left. Some guys faced it straight on and bent their butts to the crowd. Others favored a forty-five-degree approach, while the more timid tried to keep their bodies parallel with the wall. The whole ordeal could take up to two hours.

One February day in 1978 a social worker at the clap clinic asked if I would be interested in participating in a hepatitis study. They were looking for people who had never had hepatitis B. When I initially came down with hepatitis in 1976, they had told me it was hepatitis A, so I volunteered. They drew some blood, tested it for hepatitis B, and after three weeks or so told me that I had indeed been infected with hepatitis B and was therefore ineligible for the study. Nine years later, in 1987, they telephoned me again. They'd saved some of my blood from that 1978 test and wanted permission to test it for HIV. They also wanted some fresh blood. I readily agreed and made an appointment to sign forms and give another sample. When I went for the results, I already knew I was positive. That had been confirmed in 1985 when Duckus and I had taken the test. But I hadn't ever had my T cells checked, so that was the only source of concern.

I knew the T-cell counts of only three other people. Duckus, who had been diagnosed with pneumocystis, had a count of 30. Two friends from the gym who seemed very healthy had counts around 450 and 700. I knew we would eventually have population statistics that would tell us what was normal, but "normal" might vary widely from person to person. I knew it would be easier to decide what my own future T-cell counts would mean if I could compare them against both population parameters and my own past history. So even though the professionals were saying, "They didn't mean anything," I wanted the number for historical purposes. In situations new to medicine "not meaning anything" is always code for "We have not yet determined what this means."

This new research project wasn't housed in the same building as the old clap clinic, but a lot of the faces were the same. My appointment was with a friend from the gym. "I've got good news and bad news," he said. "Which do you want to know first?"

"The bad," I responded, without the slightest hesitation.

"Well, the bad you already know, so it's not really news for you. Your blood was positive for HIV."

Despite the fact that he knew that I knew, he nonetheless delivered the "bad news" with one of those open expressions that gives permission for a reaction, that even seems to hope for one. I had none. I'd been living with this for quite some time. Steve had been dead almost two years now. Duckus had already come down with pneumocystis. Now this guy whom I knew from the gym, with whom I'd had several conversations about being positive, was "giving me news." Maybe it's because he was sitting behind a desk. I guess they had a training session or something. Whatever.

"So what's the good news?"

"You were HIV negative in 1978."

"Why is that good news?" I asked. "I was hoping I was positive in 1978. That would mean I had survived this thing for nine years already, at the least."

"Because our research shows that the only thing that correlates with survival is time since infection."

"What! That's impossible. What sort of factors are you looking at? How are you collecting the data?"

"We're looking at everything. We have an incredibly sophisticated design that looks at all aspects of sexuality, drug use, psychological testing, demographic factors. We have a top team of public health professionals, epidemiologists, survey researchers, biostatisticians. I know it is not very hopeful, but that is what the research is showing. To date, the only thing that correlates with survival is the length of time since becoming infected. So it is very good that you weren't infected in 1978. It isn't uncommon for people to live with this thing for five years, and of course research continues to look for treatments."

"So what are my T cells—good or bad?"

"Well, your T cells are 714, which is high, but that really doesn't mean anything. I can't emphasize this too strongly. T-cell levels have not yet been correlated with survival. We don't know what T cells mean. Some people are living a long time with very low T cells, and some people are getting sick with relatively high T-cell counts. Not even drug use has been correlated with survival time. The sad thing is, the only thing that correlates with survival is time since getting infected."

"Yeah, right. I know they don't mean anything yet. But they will someday. What kind of qualitative data are you collecting?"

"For those who were positive in 1978–80 we're asking a lot of questions, especially about sex and drug use."

"And what about those who were negative in the early stages? Are you asking them the same questions?"

"Unfortunately, there isn't enough funding to do everything we'd like to do."

I suspected that increased funding wasn't the problem. I suspected that the entrenched methods and procedures of the public health establishment were the problem. "The reason nothing correlates with survival," I answered "is that you're probably not asking the right people the right questions. It's pretty presumptuous, don't you think, to say nothing correlates with survival just because you haven't found anything yet?"

"Well, of course, as we get more data, things might change. All of us hope something will correlate with survival. Hope is very important, but science is important, too. This is an incredibly well-designed study."

"Have you written down that I tested positive in September 1985, or is this research going to show my HIV positive test date as 1987?"

"I'll write it down if you like, but the statistics will be run on the 1987 test date. This is very rigorous scientific research, and the grant requires that we gather verifiable data. I'm sure you know when you were first tested, but as you know, many people are not reliable historians."

"My concern is that your results are not going to be reliable either. Yet you'll convince the public it's the gospel truth because you've done such good science. If you don't ask people when they tested positive, you won't ever be able to go back and run your statistics again—once for your verifiable stuff and once for what people in the community are saying—even if you do get more funding."

He indulged my harangue about this type of epidemiological work for a while, and I left the office depressed. Maybe nothing but time since infection would correlate with survival. That was really disappointing. It meant that the virus was stronger than everyone, that the virus would catch up with everyone. Survival itself lessened one's chance for survival. I didn't really know what data they were collecting or how they were analyzing it, but I was deeply suspicious. Just because science had not discovered anything that affected disease progression (other than time since infection) did not mean genetic or psychosocial correlations did not exist. However, the pronouncements of researchers were made with such conviction that even skeptics such as myself were sometimes tempted to abandon their hope.

A few months later I was having breakfast with Gabe and reading the *Chronicle*. "Jesus!" I screamed across the breakfast table. "Who do these jerks think they are? Are they just idiots or what?"

"The bit about the average survival time?" Gabe asked calmly.

"You already read it?"

"Before you got up."

"What in God's name do they mean by average? Where do they manage to find averages? They won't be able to find the mean until the last one of us drops dead. Any average calculated before that is going to be short. Any projection that they tweak from the data so far is only going to represent the ones who died first. This is just crap. Probably hundreds of thousands of dollars' worth of crap."

"Are they assuming that the group of us with HIV are distributed over some sort of bell curve?" Gabe asked, trying both to soothe my nerves and engage my rational processes.

"Probably. But that is a guess out of nowhere. The assumptions behind these statistical projections are never discussed. The survival curve for people with HIV could take a dozen different shapes, but the ones who will live the longest are clearly not comparable to those who will die first. And the people who were infected early may well not be comparable to the people who were infected five years later. And neither group may be comparable to those who are being infected today. Supposedly this virus is mutating, but even if it isn't, those who got infected in 1979 probably include a greater proportion of people with weaker immune responses to this virus. All they know is the average length of time it took for the first 30 percent to drop dead. They don't know how long it's going to take for the next 30 percent to die. They sure don't know how long it's going to take the last 30 percent to die. And by that time people will have eaten so many pharmaceuticals that they'll never be able to calculate an average survival time that means anything at all."

Later I discovered the assumptions behind their statistical methods weren't discussed in the scientific journals that published the studies either. Perhaps that was because the audience reading scientific journals already knew the theoretical assumptions behind each statistical method, so it would be redundant. Perhaps lay journalists covering medical news simply needed to be educated. But I suspected that the problem wasn't confined to journalists. Most of the American researchers in the social and medical sciences I'd met were either unable or unwilling to discuss the philosophical assumptions on which their methods were based. The doubt that used to be a hallmark of good scientific thinking had been preempted by a devotion to instruments of measurement and profitable products.

As time went on, this became less and less surprising to me. For nearly four decades now sociologists have been describing how the modern medical industry has assumed much of the authority and responsibility that used to adhere to the church. Today medical science charges dissenters such as Robert Root-Bernstein, Joseph Sonnabend, and Peter Duesberg with heresy.[1] Today medical science is the nearly indisputable arbiter of truths concerning all matters related to health and illness.

I met Matthew and his lover, Robert, at the gym in the late 1970s. To my mind they were the epitome of a successful open gay relationship. (They had been together for fifteen years when Robert died.) Both were extremely bright and very handsome. Popular, promiscuous, and successful, Robert was a brilliant economist whom I both loved and admired, and Matthew reminded me of my lover, Steve.

I interviewed Matthew because he had been HIV positive since 1978, his status having been documented because of his participation in the San Francisco hepatitis study. Thus, he was the longest documented survivor of HIV whom I knew. My closest friends and I had often theorized about what kind person might survive HIV infection. Since Matthew was our living example of a survivor, he had became a kind of lay case study and a reason to hope. I was of course interested in lifestyle and medical decisions, but what I found was a story of love, irreplaceable loss, and a reluctance to be perceived as any sort of model survivor. As soon as I turned on the tape recorder, Matthew took over.

"I'm better off answering specific questions than rambling on about my story," he began.

"Okay. When did you first—"

"Is the tape on?"

"Yeah."

"Oh. Let me fix my hair."

"When did you first hear about AIDS?" I continued, trying to take a bit of control.

"I don't know. I think I've lost my sense of time. I had a friend over last night for dinner, and he mentioned his lover had died five and a half years ago. I would have sworn it was around three years ago. If I'd thought about it, I could have figured it out by going back from when Robert got sick in 1986. It was before that. So I seem to have lost my time line. My guess is that I started hearing about it probably seven or eight years ago."

"Which would make it 1982 or 1983."

"In that general time frame. I knew relatively early because one of the first cases in the city was a friend of mine. I remember when they were diagnosing one or two cases a week, and I thought that was a lot. So it was fairly early."

"When did you take the HIV test? Was it before Robert was diagnosed?"

"No. At that point we both felt that there was no reason to take the test because you couldn't do anything about it. It just would have upset us. The city had already contacted me to say that they had blood samples of mine from 1978 and blood samples from Robert from 1979. So we knew that those were sitting there. We had a long history at the clinic and were just waiting for a reason to take the HIV test. About a month after Robert was diagnosed with KS [Kaposi's sarcoma],[2] we left for Europe for two months. When we came back, I had the test."

"What was it like to get the test results? Was it hard?"

"It was very difficult because there's always a chance that you're negative, even though you assume you're positive. One reason you don't get tested is that you think there's a chance that you're negative. I had a friend whose lover had died of AIDS, yet he tested negative. But my reaction to being positive wasn't as bad as it could have been. If I had gone in and been told I was positive, I think it would have felt like the earth was moving and the floor was falling out from under me. But I was basically told, 'You're positive, and you've been positive since 1978.' So I was already positive for quite a number of years."

"What did that mean to you? How did you interpret that?"

"I interpreted that as a good sign. At that point they didn't really know what the incubation period was, but they were talking about two to three years. I was well beyond that, so I figured it was a good sign. I would have been more concerned if I hadn't been positive in 1978. I felt better having all those years under me. As it turns out, I don't feel better about it now, because they've just changed the incubation period to eleven years."

"Eleven and a half—they change it every year."

"Yeah. They keep raising it. I thought that I was past the incubation period, but it's just not happening that way. I'm at twelve and a half years now."

▼▼▼

Matthew was not the only person who was disappointed by the news that the average length of time from infection to AIDS was increasing. When he got tested in 1986, being HIV positive since 1978 seemed to mean he had a high chance of being in the group that might "survive." In 1990 when this interview was conducted, the expanded average time from infection to AIDS (from around five years to eleven years) meant that he was only one year beyond the average. What should have been interpreted as good news for HIV-positive people became bad news for those who had always striven to be as far "above" the norm as possible, whether in terms of grades, sports competitions, or salaries. With HIV, death had defined the norm from the beginning. Even after the virus failed to kill all of its victims in the monolithic fashion that the experts expected, even when the predicted "average" survival time increased from five to eleven-plus years, death still defined the norm. To beat death, we had to somehow beat the average, and the average time had grown so long that it was impossible to beat.

For Matthew, this annual change said the same thing it did to several men in my community: "This is your year to die. We thought it was last year, but we were wrong. It's this year." Whether from AIDS researchers' inflated sense of self-importance or from the media's uncritical faith in their utterances, a measure of cruelty emanated from those reports that affected even those of us who doubted them from the beginning. Several men in this study were angry about those projections, not so much because they were so far from the truth, but because they were swallowed whole by the mainstream press. If the press moved just a few of its political pundits to the biomedical beat, the modicum of doubt, skepticism, and alternative thinking kept alive in our political discourse might produce a revolution in America's thinking about sickness and health. In fact, academic thinking is way behind what people are practicing. One-third of Americans already use alternative medical practitioners.[3]

▼ ▼ ▼

"So you've been positive since 1978. You found out in 1986. When did you start measuring T cells?"

"In 1986. As long as I was positive, I wanted to know what was going on, so I started measuring T cells. They've always been in the same range, between 500 and 600. There was one test that was way higher than that, and I just assumed that it was a fluke, not an accurate test."

"Have you done anything in terms of lifestyle changes or anything as a result of being positive or having 500 or 600 T cells."

"It's not that I have 500 or 600 T cells. I think I would have made the same changes if they were 700 or 800. I started taking acyclovir four years ago because I thought that AIDS was eventually going to be associated with herpes.[4] I'd never had it, so I figured, Why bother getting herpes? My doctor said it wasn't harmful, and I felt like I was doing something, so I've been taking acyclovir since 1986. I've tried various things. I took that muck you put in the blender, AL-721. I did that for about a year. I've tried various things. I still do acyclovir, and I started AZT two months ago."

"Tell me about the acyclovir first. How much do you take?"

"It varies. At different times I've been on different amounts, from as many as ten a day to as few as three a day. At the moment I'm on six a day. I'm taking six AZTs, so I thought six would keep it simple."

"Does your physician have any recommendation on how much acyclovir you should take? Has he given you any sort of range?"

"His recommendation is none. He really doesn't think it makes much difference if I take three or four or five or six. He was more comfortable with six than ten, but he lets me participate. I figure it's my decision since it's my body."

"So you took acyclovir to prevent herpes. Why did you take AL-721?"

"Well, the initial reports on AL-721 looked promising. It was totally nontoxic, and I figured, Why not do it as long as there are no side effects, other than being inconvenient? Things come out and you hear great things about them, and then you hear nothing else about them ever again, and you figure, well, they must not have found anything. I didn't see anything negative about it—except that it didn't do anything. But I never saw anything positive about it again."

"I read a report that said people taking it had fewer night sweats and less thrush, but that it didn't change T cells and had no effect on the immune system. I stopped taking it, too, even though I thought the conclusion of the study that debunked it was crap. Egg lecithin doesn't kill thrush by itself. It has to affect the immune system. They're all looking for a cure, and AL-721 wasn't a cure. I think we all stopped taking it at about the same time.

"What about going on AZT?" I continued. "How did you decide to do that?"

"My decision about that was from the research coming out. They only get T cells within a range, so there's no real difference between 525 and 475. My doctor seemed to think that when you get below 500, you should start AZT. They have an attitude of 'when, not if.' It's like they're waiting. It's sort of creeping up on you. I figure as long as it's going to be eventual—and they keep telling me it's eventual, that it's going to happen, that they're going to drop another 25 or another 10 or whatever—I might as well just start it now."

"What were your physician's arguments?"

"For not taking the AZT? There's no research done above 500, no statistics to show that it does anything. The only studies were in the 200 to 500 level. Granted, it was significant, but the sample was so small that he didn't consider it relevant. But I disagree. I know a number of people who are taking AZT and have had dramatic increases in their T cells, which I find strange."

"Is it like the acyclovir? You just feel like you should be doing something?"

"Well, it's not just feeling that I should be doing something. I have this horrible feeling that at some point we'll find out that this is what you should have been doing all along, and now it's too late. You should have been doing this two years ago or whatever. I guess I figure I should do something. AZT is all that's out there at the moment that's approved, and it seems to be relatively nontoxic or relatively safe. I had a friend who was just killed by ddI—from pancreatic failure.[5] I don't have those worries about AZT. Since I've started taking it, I had my blood work done again this week, and my red and white cells are fine. The doctor said that my white cells were up and so were my red cells."

"So you're obviously not getting anemic from it. You said you've been on it for two months?"

"Yeah."

"Have you had any side effects?"

"I get tired in the middle of the afternoon, and I seem to urinate at night. I have to get up to go to the bathroom three or four times."

"What do you do when you're tired in the middle of the afternoon?"

"Lie down usually."

"Do you sleep?"

"Not usually. Sometimes a little bit. If I sleep, it's like fifteen minutes or something. One day when I was in Florida in a shopping mall with my mother, I had to sit down because otherwise I was going to keel over. I've gotten that tired a couple of times."

"When you say you felt like you were going to keel over, what do you mean?"

"I felt like I was just going to fall asleep. I was that tired."

"Did you feel a little light-headed?"

"No more than usual," he said, laughing. "I just felt tired—and heavy—like my body had to go down. The other side effect is that I seem to have not a great deal of interest in sex, which is highly unusual for me. I'll have a date over, and instead of having sex, we'll watch TV and I'll fall asleep. Or the other night the guy I've been dating was out of town. About 10:30 I was going to go down to Folsom Street to party at the 890 (a sex club), but I thought I'd rather go to sleep. Sounded like more fun. So I went to sleep."

"Are there any other things you feel like you're not doing because you're HIV positive?"

"I don't think so. I pretty much do what I want. I look at other people, and they have all kinds of other difficulties. I don't have any financial problems. I'm able to busy myself, to buy houses, and to do what I want. I don't worry about getting sick most of the time, but I don't want to put myself in a situation where I'm in the middle of something and then get sick. If I weren't worried about getting sick, I would have built a new house instead of buying a new house. I'd like an estate on eighty or one hundred acres, with a caretaker's house and a guest house to get people out from under my nose when they're there. I would have built a relatively simple house—by my standards, which I guess wouldn't be all that simple. But I couldn't see being in the middle of construction and then getting sick."

"Have you made any changes with drugs or alcohol?"

"My drug use was always less significant than people thought it was. I didn't really do that many drugs. Robert liked poppers. I didn't give up grass and I won't. I don't do it that often, and it's not a big deal."

Matthew took care of himself by doing what he wanted to when he wanted to. When he got tired, he napped; he stopped. His immediate feeling or state of mind was far more important than meeting some preestablished expectations, his own or those of others. Even when he planned a date or a trip to a sex club, if his attitude or energy changed, he went with it.

Matthew was also a man who thought things through for himself. He generally accepted the medical establishment's appraisal of the situation: "They have an attitude of when, not if," and he decided to begin using pharmaceuticals early. His explanation for taking acyclovir and AZT before his physician recommended it had nothing to do with needing hope, power, or control. Matthew understood himself as having power and control already. Rather his attitude was expressed in very pragmatic terms: "I figure as long as it's going to be eventual—and they keep telling me it's eventual . . . I might as well just start it now." Although Matthew organized much of his story around the loss of his lover, Robert, he didn't tell it in terms of having to make changes or give things up.

"Once Robert was diagnosed and we got over the initial shock, things didn't change much. The major change was that Robert wasn't going to work anymore. He went on disability and was home all the time. After three or four months had gone by and he seemed fine and nothing happened, AIDS just became something to live with. For at least a year I really didn't think in terms of Robert's getting any sicker or about anything further than the moment. You never know. Some people just go on. Then about two years after he was diagnosed, we noticed some changes in his health."

"So for two years you tried hard to just kind of deny it?"

"I don't think we were denying it. The previous idea was that you got AIDS and you died. People all around us were dying, and that was a constant reminder. But the new idea developing was that you have AIDS and you live with it. After being diagnosed, AIDS was our life. But then life went on. Then when Robert got sick, AIDS became our life again."

"What has sex been like since AIDS or since Robert was diagnosed?"

"At first we stopped having sex with other people. We had been fairly promiscuous. I remember when I went to something or other and they asked me what I missed the most about sex in the old days, and my answer was, 'Being called a slut and taking it as a compliment.' We didn't know many people with AIDS at first. Then we called someone up to have sex with, and the person had been diagnosed two days earlier. At that point we both stopped having sex with other people.

"Another change was rubbers. We hadn't been using rubbers with each other. We figured we'd been having sex for ten years together without rubbers and if we'd exposed each other, we'd exposed each other and that's the way it is. After Robert was diagnosed, one of the doctors said that repeated exposure may not be good, so we started using rubbers with each other. Robert liked them less than I do. Then about a year after he was diagnosed, I started having sex with other people again, and I just assumed everybody was positive. That was my attitude. It was always very, very safe. It slacks up a little sometimes, but I think it's still within safe-sex guidelines, from beating off to intercourse. But intercourse is always with rubbers, and I don't believe in cumming in a rubber. I think there's too much potential to tear.

"I realize that on the spectrum of things, everybody's idea of 'safe' is different, and some people would say that I'm being very safe, and others would say I'm not being safe enough. My guess is that if I were negative, I would probably have a different set of guidelines. I'm not comfortable going out with people who think they are negative. I figure they may be negative, they may not be negative, but I don't want anyone to feel that I'm responsible for making them positive. So I prefer going out with someone who's positive."

"You mentioned also that about a year after Robert was diagnosed, you started having sex with other people. What was that about? How did that work for the two of you?"

"It just sort of happened. It was no big deal. Robert wasn't much interested in sex, and I still was. Robert became interested in sex only with certain people, and he was interested in doing things that I wasn't into. He had a couple of little sex friends, and most of my sex was like at the 1808 Club, you know, beating off and stuff.

"AIDS can bring people together or pull them apart. After a while Robert just developed other interests. He had his spiritual people and his crystals and things that I did not share an interest in. It didn't create friction to have different interests. It just created a separation. My feeling is that whatever one believes, if it helps them, then that's good. But some of the stuff with psychics got to be a bit much for me. We went to this thing in Palo Alto where there was another voice going through the body and stuff. I figured they were profiteering off a lot of us, and I got annoyed with it. It's one thing to have Lazarus, but it's another thing to have Lazarus stores.[6] Robert would tell me that Lazarus wasn't the one profiteering; it was the channel. You'd think that Lazarus would speak to the channel and tell them not to profiteer. Robert could certainly afford it, but I had friends who had limited resources and were spending their money on this.

"But people explore until they find what fits. Robert went into each thing with gusto and picked up pieces of each thing that worked for him. Some things worked better than others, and he stuck with them. He took what he could from things that didn't really work and just combined them into his little patchwork of whatever was going to help. I had interest in some things and doubts about others. Some of it seemed totally ridiculous. It was difficult at times for me to not share that with him, which was not being very supportive, but I could only go so far with some of it.

"I almost felt like I lost Robert about six months before he died. There was suddenly this wedge between us that wasn't there before. I felt I was there as a caretaker. There was an emotional change maybe four or five months before he died, but I was aware of it before his final illness. I withdrew a little bit. There's probably still something that hasn't come out. I don't know. I had very little in the way of tears after he died. I was just sort of numb for a while. I think a lot of it was just pushed out of my mind.

"I still have Robert in the box upstairs. I haven't opened it, and I'm reluctant to part with it. I was going to take some of his ashes to Italy and some to the country, but I figured, well, I don't want to have him all over different places. How would he get back together again? I find it strange that I'm keeping the box of ashes there. I used to keep it out on the bathroom counter, but yesterday I put it away, under the counter. I was straightening up, and I figured it had been there for two months. When I was in the other house, I didn't want it in the closet because it was dark. I find it all a little peculiar."

"I haven't scattered Duckus's ashes. If I ever do, it will be in one place."

"Why?"

"I think that that's what he would want. Yet he never told me exactly what to do with them."

"Robert didn't care. He was quite specific that he didn't care what happened to them. I thought I might take a cup of it and dump it in the river in Florence—or someplace—but who knows."

"I don't know where to put Duckus because I don't know where I'm going to put me. Do you ever think about that?"

"No, because I haven't decided what will happen to me. I don't know that I want to be cremated. I may want to go into the family plot. On the other hand, being underground sounds so unappealing. But I don't want to be burned either."

"Being underground goes on and on and on. At least the burning is fast," I laughed. "It's all quite weird."

"I'll tell you what bothers me, and it's way off. I can't believe that they've not come up with a term for a deceased lover. You'd think with all the creative minds—the theatrical, verbal, spiritual minds—that there'd be some sort of term. When I talk about Robert, I don't want to call him my former lover. I feel funny referring to him as my deceased lover. I really don't know how to refer to him when I talk about him, and I've talked to other people who have lost their lovers, and they all feel the same way. There's no word for it. Wouldn't you imagine that someone would come up with that?"

"What does the heterosexual community use? Do they have such words? They don't. I don't think they do."

"But you're referred to as a widow or a widower. There's not even a word for that for us. It's not really correct to be considered a widower. I just don't feel comfortable with that. We need something that's not masculine/feminine, something 'nondenominational.' How do you refer to Duckus?"

"As my lover. Then I have to explain that he's gone. It's weird. It's always awkward."

"It's awkward for the other person because then you have to explain that they've died. It's socially awkward, and it's emotionally awkward, which I think is more important."

"What's dating been like since Robert died?"

"I think another relationship is improbable. I think I'll date people. Once I thought about whether I'd like to live with someone I was dating, but then I thought, no. By the time you hit forty, you have your home, your friends, and your own way of doing things. Then suddenly there's someone new. In the old days you did things together. You bought a house, you furnished an apartment together, you made friends together. I have all that stuff now, and the last thing I'd want is someone moving in here who didn't have my taste. I know, bad taste is really just taste that isn't my taste. If their taste is too good, it's bad to me. The right amount of funk, the right amount of this. I'm looking for me. So I think that seems improbable."

"That you'll find somebody like you?"

"It's not really me because I wouldn't go out with me, but someone who has interests that are similar enough, taste that is overlapping enough, all that type of stuff. I think that seems improbable. The people that I go out with seem to be less sophisticated than I would like. That's an elitist attitude, but you spend twenty years looking at art, going to the ballet and the opera, analyzing films, whatever, or just looking at things with a certain analytical eye. Then you meet someone who's very nice, and they've spent that time in the discos. It's just a difference in experience and what you see when you're with someone. I could go with Robert to some little town in the middle of nowhere, and we'd find things that were absolutely awe-inspiring. We could sit and look at the stonework in a wall for an hour—just a bunch of rocks piled up three hundred years ago—and see something in it and appreciate it. How do you find that again? Someone else might say, 'Gee that's a nice wall.'

"When we'd take trips, we wouldn't want to just be everywhere at once, so we'd try to get a focus. We'd focus fairly arbitrarily. One year we decided that what we were interested in were floor patterns. We were in various cathedrals in Italy, and everybody was looking at the stained glass windows, and we're photographing the floors. It's hard to do this with other people."

"You mentioned a support group. Have you ever felt a need to get involved in a group that dealt with grief issues, especially in terms of Robert?"

"Well, in my Friday group we devoted a meeting to my grief. That's the thing to do. But I haven't gone to one of their grief groups. I think my grief is something private, and I don't think it would help me to sit with a bunch of strangers and talk about my grief. In order to understand my grief, you'd have to know me and you'd have to know Robert."

▼ ▼ ▼

There were a number of issues that created a sense of loss for Matthew before Robert died. They had a long history of supporting each other's divergent interests, but Robert's diagnosis brought these differences into stark relief. There was a wedge between them that hadn't been there before. Part of that wedge was certainly due to changing sexual and spiritual interests, but part of it was due to the simple fact of Robert's getting sicker. Matthew tried to support Robert's new directions, but that attempt came from his new role as a caregiver, not out of the long-term relationship they had enjoyed together.

Matthew was well aware that AIDS brought some people closer and pushed others apart, but a "big picture" awareness did not end his story. Matthew did not need information or processes. He knew what was going on inside himself. Matthew's grief was private. This is something health professionals and academicians must take seriously. The movement to capture the most fundamental aspects of our humanity in concepts, precise definitions, and universal social interventions often does more for academic careers than it does to relieve human suffering or develop better understandings of the human condition. Talking about grief is not the same as grieving. Sharing stories of deep personal loss with a therapeutic community of strangers is a modern invention that does not work for everyone. Although professional strangers are certainly necessary in modern times, they are no substitute for a community where life is celebrated and death is shared. Even when mourning is shared, the most profound grief is both private and universal, but rarely social.

Matthew also saw his long-term asymptomatic status as something personal and refused to help me develop a theoretical understanding of surviving HIV.

▼ ▼ ▼

"I'd like to share some of my own impressions about how you are dealing with all of this, to see what you think of them. I know that a newspaper would say that you're average—that you've lived the average amount of time since being HIV positive. Of course, as you keep living longer, they keep upping the average. But never mind what the statisticians are saying about the future. You're the longest surviving HIV-positive person we know about. So I'm pretending that I'm an anthropologist going to those places where people live to be 110 and asking them what the secret of their longevity is."

"I don't like that. A couple of years ago someone said, 'You're the kind of person who gives us hope because we see that you've been positive all these years and you seem to be fine.' It's a responsibility I'm not real thrilled about. I have the feeling that if I get sick, it's going to wreck all these people. I figure it would be enough for me to be sick without worrying about how everyone else might react. I could imagine people coming over and not being sure if they were concerned about me or about themselves."

"I can understand that, but right now you have managed for a long time with this, and our community needs to paint profiles of survivors. Whether you get sick or not, at this point you're still in the survival mode. Gabe and I were talking about survival last week. You're not the only one, but we used you and a couple of other people to generate some initial thoughts about what it might take to survive this thing. I think you are an interesting model for survival because you're one of those people that combines a lot of opposites. You care about other people but are totally self-obsessed. You are as anxious as anyone, but you know about what help is available. You look at it all and don't really believe in any of it. Skeptical, yet engaged. It's almost a kind of healthy neurosis that's not about denial or acceptance or belief. You seem to be walking this very fine line. It's not about repressing a huge amount of feelings; it's not about giving vent to all the feelings. You're this odd combination of responses to—"

"Then how come I can't get a good date?"

Matthew neither confirmed nor denied the analysis Gabe and I had constructed to explain why someone might survive with HIV. Matthew was not interested in our theories of survival and changed the subject with one of his typical wisecracks. And whereas Matthew's story revolved around the loss of Robert, it cannot be adequately framed or interpreted with psychosocial concepts such as grief, social support, hope, or fear. To know Matthew's loss, you had to know Matthew, and what emerged most clearly from his story was an incredibly strong sense of self.

But Matthew's story was not simply a collection of idiosyncratic concerns. Losing people before they died or deciding what to do with a loved one's ashes reflects wider cultural concerns that become increasingly relevant as lesbians and gay men establish new identities, families, communities, and traditions. Matthew was vitally interested in community and participated in programs that lent support to people with AIDS. He never blamed the dominant culture for failing to develop effective treatments or for denying us a language in which to express our love and our grief. He was a part of that dominant culture and simply asked why the smarter members of our community had not already invented the language we needed.

Likewise, decision-making theory does help us understand Matthew's choice about early intervention with AZT. Matthew was certainly aware of a possible downside to taking AZT too early, but his decision was not framed as a rational cost-benefit analysis. Rather, he expressed it in terms of the mistake he did not want to make—waiting too long before taking advantage of something that would have helped. Nor was his story primarily about hopes or fears. For instance, Matthew seemed less overtly fearful than Nathan, but also less overtly hopeful. As much as possible, Matthew even avoided casting the lifestyle changes he made during the 1980s in terms of HIV. Instead, matters such as reducing recreational drug use were presented as outcomes of his own personal development, his own changing desires.

Despite the fact that the numbers keep pushing him closer to the norm, Matthew remains one of our longest known survivors, having tested positive in 1978. Twenty years later, in 1998, Matthew still has not developed AIDS. Perhaps it is good that he rejected the poster boy role. The new research protocols don't count him as a long-term survivor anyway. He doesn't meet the new criteria for a "long-term nonprogressor." Almost none of us does. We don't have enough T cells.

| 5 |

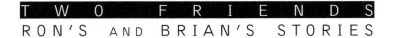

RON'S AND BRIAN'S STORIES

There are certainly many gay men whose understandings of health, illness, and HIV are largely consistent with those of the dominant culture. Their stories have been told in a number of books—Emmanuel Dreuilhe's *Mortal Embrace*, Hervé Guibert's *To the Friend Who Did Not Save My Life*, Paul Monette's *Borrowed Time*, and David Feinberg's *Queer and Loathing*. In those stories people with AIDS joined with their physicians to war against disease. Theories about health and illness were not the major issues in that body of work. People who were suffering needed to get whatever help and comfort were available, often regardless of beliefs. But for asymptomatics, beliefs about health and illness were more central and often drove decisions about how to manage HIV.

Like Nathan and Matthew, the two stories told here reflect strong beliefs in the products of Western medicine. Whereas Nathan at first resisted AZT and the drugs that initially made him feel sick, he eventually embraced the new antivirals wholeheartedly. Matthew wanted to make sure he didn't wait too long before taking AZT. Ron shared those concerns, and both he and his friend Brian embraced AZT. But Ron's and Brian's experiences with the medical establishment went beyond drugs and blood tests. For Ron, the health care system functioned as an authority structure that could foster either hope or despair. Brian often bypassed the system, preferring to get the most sensitive information from a friend who was a physician.

Unlike most stigmatized people, Ron and Brian were not excluded from the rituals and sacraments that constitute the dominant culture's healing and caring practices. In San Francisco gay men were not as alienated from the traditional structures of help as they are in many other places. Nonetheless, both of their stories demonstrate how subtle forms of alienation can thrive even within largely supportive communities.

Fervent Belief: Ron

I knew Ron and his lover of many years, James, from the gym. Both of them were very buffed muscle queens who were sweet, outgoing, and easy on the eyes. They were both HIV positive.

After finishing a torturous abdominal workout one Saturday afternoon, I went to see whether Ron was almost finished with his Stair-Master. He'd worked up a major sweat but still had energy enough to chatter away at me for his last three minutes. By the time he was finished, I discovered that his "society" AIDS doctor was treating him "aggressively" with dextran sulfate and a Chinese herbal formula called Resist and that he attributed his asymptomatic status and relatively high T-cell count to those interventions. We agreed to meet at his house at 10:00 the next morning to continue the conversation on tape. Neither of us expected to be out very late.

James was watching TV with their friend Brian in the den, and we settled into the living room. After a bit of coffee and chitchat we returned to the topics from the day before. Ron had been tested in 1987, and I asked what made him decide to do it.

▼ ▼ ▼

"It was because my ex-lover came down with AIDS. I'd met him about ten and a half years ago, in 1979. I'd been more sexually active with him on a continual basis than anybody in my life. It was totally unsafe sex. We didn't know anything about unsafe sex other than going for regular VD checks."

"Was he the first person you'd been sexually involved with who came down with AIDS?"

"No. Other people I had been sexually involved with had been diagnosed, but those relationships were so far in the past. I don't know if they passed anything on to me or not—or if I passed anything on to them. I know now that I was still negative in 1980 because the VD clinic did a hepatitis study ten years ago. They phoned to ask if they could unfreeze my sample and test it for HIV. I told them they didn't need to test it because I already knew that I was HIV positive, but they tested it anyway and said I was negative ten years ago."

"We had the test around '85, and you had it done around '87. Why did you wait?"

"There was no known treatment. They'd just tell you to clean up your act with safe sex. I was practicing safe sex anyway because I didn't want to infect anybody, and if I wasn't infected, I didn't want to get infected. I always knew that drinking and drugs and late nights and all that kind of stuff was bad for you. I'd already started to cut that stuff out, clean up my act, and lead a clean, healthy life. Since there wasn't any treatment, I figured, Why get upset? If I can go through life feeling more optimistic, that can only make me feel better. But the minute I found out through James that AZT was around and was effective for treatment, we both decided to go down and take the test. We didn't want to take AZT unless we were actually positive. But the minute we knew there was some kind of positive action we could take, besides just living a good clean life, then it made sense to take the test. I figured that finding out I was positive wouldn't be such a disaster since there was something I could do about it.

"I never had much doubt in my mind. I figured I maybe had a 10 or 20 percent chance of being negative. I was surprised when I found out certain other people were positive, but I wasn't surprised about myself. I wasn't happy about it, but I wasn't surprised."

"What was it like for you?"

"I think I would've been okay, but two things scared me to death. First, they sat me down at the clinic to give me the results and were so heavy about it that it scared me. Then they suggested that I go to a support group at Project Inform. That turned out to be the most horrible experience of my life. It was about twenty or thirty people who all sat around and talked about how great life was before AIDS and that they would all be dead in a year. So instead of being supported, I ended up cheering everybody up. I felt good about that. But it was a bunch of defeatist people sitting around saying things like, 'It's over; how am I going to tell my parents or my mother that I'm positive, that I'm going to be getting sicker and sicker, that they're going to have to take care of me?' The whole feeling was death. There wasn't one person in the group who was thinking that they'd make it, that they might live a normal life span and not ever come down with AIDS or ARC. Except for me. That was one of the worst experiences I've gone through since the day that I found out that I was almost going to be drafted through the lottery.

"When I told my doctor about the support group, he was horrified. He said he wished I hadn't gone, but the people at the clinic practically forced me to go. They made it sound like it was standard procedure and that it would be really helpful. They made me feel like if I didn't do it, I wouldn't be doing everything possible to help myself. The whole testing procedure up to that point was fine."

"It sounds like the counselor was too caught up in his own feelings about HIV to appreciate where you were coming from."

"They could've handled it differently. They sat me down like it was the biggest thing in my life and made me feel like everyone they tested in the last several weeks came up negative. I really got the impression that they were singling me out. I sort of went in knowing I was going to be positive. I went out totally broken.

"I went to see my best friend because James was at work, and he made me feel better. Then by the end of the evening I felt fine—until I started going to that group three to four days later, and then it was horrible. They made you do meditation and all that kind of stuff, and I'm not into that. Then I felt guilty because I'm not into meditation and self-healing and all that stuff. I'm a kind of a real medical person. I would've preferred their saying that they're doing this research and they have this drug and that drug. Even if it wasn't true, that would have made me feel better. You're supposed to go like once a week, but I just went one day. It scared the hell out of me, and I never went back. And from that moment on I felt better and better and better."

▼▼▼

Some have argued that medical information is never neutral and that the metaphors surrounding AIDS have been as deadly as the virus. This is an interesting position in light of Ron's reaction to the HIV test. Ron had approached the HIV test within a context of hope and care. As a medically sanctioned intervention, AZT provided the impetus and the courage for him to take the test, but that was not the context in which Ron was received. Neither the counselor nor the people at the Project Inform meeting shared Ron's faith and hope in Western medicine. The psychosocial-spiritual interventions they offered in its place were as comforting to Ron as a bottle of AZT would have been to those who believed it was poison.

Ron's experience reversed the usual state of affairs. Usually, it is the medicalized, rather than the psychosocial, understanding of health and the body that is crammed down people's throats. Ron's experience shows that health care providers of all persuasions can impose their own values and expectations onto unwilling patients. Ron believed in Western medicine, and he responded to the counselor's authority as a health professional. Ron was "made to feel" that if he did not go to the support group, he was not doing everything possible to help himself. Ron did not simply react to the support group by getting angry or bored or by dismissing the whole thing as utter nonsense. He responded with horror and guilt. He felt guilty for not liking meditation while feeling forced to do it. Even those of us who, unlike Ron, adopt a critical, analytical stance with our health care providers cannot altogether avoid similar experiences. When people seek help from socially sanctioned health authorities, their vulnerability must confront one of the most powerful and intimidating professional bureaucracies of our time. Those who reject the dominant interpretations of their illnesses often endure thinly veiled insinuations of blame and stupidity from their health care providers. Fortunately, Ron had a physician who lent authoritative weight to his decision not to go back. After a while Ron and James became dissatisfied with the standard research-confirmed medical practice offered by this same physician and decided to go to a medical clinic with a reputation for treating HIV more aggressively.

"James mentioned an HIV clinic offering aggressive medical treatment for asymptomatics. Then I saw an advertisement for the clinic in a gay magazine, and I thought maybe it was real sleazy. But James had heard about it from friends. Then my father's sister, who's a brain surgeon at Stanford, checked into it, and we decided to go.

"After my first appointment I felt a thousand times better. These people were saying that we didn't have to die from AIDS and research is showing that there are treatments for it—maybe not cures, but treatments. They were doing things that were more radical, like putting people on AZT when their T-cell count was 400 when other doctors were using it at 200 or less. Everything they've come up with has become more standard practice.[1] They're very optimistic. Several doctors there are HIV positive. That makes me feel better because I know that this guy is in the same boat as I am. He's not some straight doctor who doesn't have a fear about getting AIDS himself.

"They were more radical with James's treatment because his T-cell count was lower than mine. I saw him improve very quickly, and he has stayed improved for a year and a half to two years. They got his T cells out of the danger zone into the normal zone. They had been 240 or less. He also went to the doctor because he had shingles on his face. That was the first sign for either of us because up to that point we were both asymptomatic. His shingles cleared up, his herpes outbreaks decreased, and his general health improved. His T-cell count is in the upper 400s and has been staying there for two years. So it's almost doubled.

"Mine's gone down a lot because my doctor wasn't doing as aggressive treatment, but it never went below 400. It's been staying in the 400–500 range. I don't seem to deteriorate, and it seems to be stabilizing. I keep mentioning that I want to go on AZT, but they don't want to put me on it. For me at this stage, they think the detrimental effects would be bigger than the positive ones. They're hoping that other medications will come out that will be better, like that ddI. They tell me the longer you can wait, the better."

"So what did you go on?"

"Just dextran sulfate—2400 mg a day. I've been doing that for almost two years. For the first six months I had no side effects at all. Then all of a sudden I got horrible diarrhea and cramps practically overnight. I'd be up five to six times a night. For days I couldn't even sleep. I got tested for everything and nothing came out positive, and I was getting sicker and sicker. Then my T-cell count dropped 200 to around 490, and I got really frightened. It turned out that I had some kind of stomach infection. He gave me some kind of drug that I took for eight days, and the cramps went away. He also took me off the dextran sulfate for three months just to make sure it wasn't that. Then he put me on something called Resist, a Chinese herb, and my T-cell count went back up a bit."

"When did you first do T cells?"

"In 1987 they were 800 or 900. But then I went to another lab, and it was 700 or 800. When I had the infection, it all of a sudden dropped to 490. When the infection cleared up, it went up to 510. That wasn't a big rise, but it was the first time it went up. It had gone down every other time I'd been tested over a few years. Then I took it again, and it went up to 536, plus some other factors besides T-cell counts improved. Again, it's nothing drastic, but twice in a row it's gone up and not down."

"Infections can take a big toll."

"I just felt awful. I didn't lose too much weight, probably ten pounds or less, but I ate a lot. The more I lost, the more I ate. But I was tired all the time because I couldn't sleep through the night. So he put me on the Chinese herb."

"Are they expensive?"

"Not when you consider—well, it's all out of my pocket. They come in bottles of 180, and a bottle is about $40 and lasts about a month. But health insurance doesn't cover it, and you add that to the dextran sulfate, which costs at least an extra $100 a month and then the huge co-pays for the doctor's office visits. It's like adding a couple of hundred dollars extra to the rent.

"I'm not so worried about dying, but about outliving my money. I'm just wondering how people can afford to take positive steps. James pays a lot more than I do. He takes a shot every two weeks, and they're $95 a shot. Then you've got to pay for those office visits, and the health insurance is getting worse and worse. Blue Shield is trying to weed out AIDS patients. They can't weed you out individually, so they tell everybody they're going to raise the deductible and premium at the end of the year. Then they come back and say, 'We have another group you can go into, but you have to reapply.' Of course, they're not going to accept you because of preexisting conditions. A nice little gimmick. It's sad. I think the big worry in the future for most people is not staying healthy, but being able to afford to stay healthy. It's going to be serious. They have treatments now, but you can't put them on your insurance. Now they're starting to hassle us for doing lab tests every quarter. The forms come back saying, 'Justify all these tests.' They haven't denied it, but they're starting to hassle people about it."

"So you submit it all back to your insurance company?"

"Yes, but my deductible went up. Originally, I was in a group where you could go to any doctor, any hospital. They paid 80 percent. They had a separate plan that was less expensive, but you had to go to certain doctors and certain hospitals to get the full benefit. Preferred providers. James went with that originally, but I could afford to go on the major benefit one. I signed up, and the first trick they did was assign me to a different group. They said, 'We're not going to change your premium, but we're going to raise your deductible, and now you've got to go to certain doctors.' If I wanted to go to any doctor, I had to reapply. Unfortunately, the doctor we want to see is not willing to be a preferred provider because he won't charge what they consider to be reasonable. U.C. Med Center is a 'preferred provider,' and they're not lousy. And several of my other doctors are preferred providers. They all agree to charge the normal and customary fees. But this clinic we go to charges a lot more. I think they're ripping us off.

"The normal visit is $75, but Blue Shield says normal visits should only be $55, and since he's not a preferred provider, they will only pay 50 percent. So for a $75 office visit, they're paying $22.50, after we reach our $750 deductible. Then on top of that, James's shots cost $95 apiece and Blue Shield won't pay at all because they don't recognize that as standard procedure. It all adds up. The dextran sulfate is $100 a month or more. Your average person can't afford it because they've still got to pay the rent. There are a lot of people around town who can't afford it, and I don't think all doctors know what they're doing. You can't go to just any old doctor or clinic. I really think you have a much better chance of living a healthy life if you can afford to go to the better doctors. I can afford it so far. I'm doing all right. But people like James! James just got a new job, and he makes just a minimal-type salary. His parents have been helping him out with money, and so have I. He works full-time. It's not like he's lazy. But what would he do if his parents and I weren't around to help him? He just wouldn't be able to afford to go to the doctor we go to."

"So what happens in the office visit with your doctor? You think he might be a rip-off?"

"I have confidence in him. You get what you pay for. You can get a haircut and pay $6 for it, or you can go to a salon and pay $35 to be pampered, and you probably get a better haircut, too. You have to decide whether it's worth it, what you can afford. You know, you go in and they weigh you and take your temp and pulse and your blood pressure. Then the doctor comes in and pulls out the chart and reads the result of your tests. And that's the end of it."

"He doesn't check your mouth or lymph nodes?"

"Well, sometimes. One good thing is that he'll ask you how you're feeling, and he'll let you ask as many questions as you want. So I figure if I'm going to get $75 worth, I sit there and ask him every question I can. We'll discuss the latest things in AIDS research. He's very informative, and he doesn't hurry, but if I didn't ask any questions, I'd be out of there in five minutes."

"So it's not that he's doing what you consider to be an excellent physical exam or anything. You mostly go to him because he's up on the research and he's willing to experiment?"

"Exactly. I've been lucky enough to be healthy since I've been going there, so there's not much he needs to do with me. I'm not really saying it's a rip-off. These are high-society doctors, and the reason I go to them is that I really do trust them. They've had hundreds of patients who are HIV positive. That's the only kind of patients they're taking—people who have not ever developed AIDS or ARC. They probably have more experience than any doctor around. I like the fact that my doctor is also HIV positive and seems to be doing quite well. All the treatments they started a year or two ago, other doctors are starting just about now."

"Do you talk to any of their other patients?"

"Oh, yeah. Almost all the guys I know who go to them are on AZT. Almost everybody that's ever gone there is on AZT, but whenever I ask anyone about their T-cell counts, they are always a lot lower than mine. My doctor told me the other day that he has several patients like me who are just doing the dextran sulfate and Resist, and their T-cell counts are not dropping. They're staying in the safe area and doing well. He wants to continue us on these because we seem to be responding to it.

"I still tend to believe that it's better to do something—better safe than sorry. I'm not the kind of person that wants to stick his head in the sand and say it may or may not affect me. I'd rather say it may not affect me, but I'm not going to take the chance."

"Do you pay attention to any other numbers besides your absolute T-cell count?"

"Well, the doctor does, and James does. I don't really understand it all and don't know if I really want to. I figure if I'm going to pay him, I'll let him do that work for me. He looks at my platelets and certain ratios, and he explains it all to me. He doesn't stress one count more than the other. I don't really know what it all means. It's like when you get your car fixed and they start explaining it all to you and showing you the parts. I figure, well, I'll just trust you; that's fine. James asked me to bring home my sheet one time, so I gave it to him. We don't discuss it too much. If it's going well, we just say it's fine; if it's going bad, we'll discuss it. It seems to be going well for both of us.

"My doctor seems to do every test in the world. They take about five vials of blood and that's part of the problem. That's why the health insurance people are starting to get on our backs. They think that he's testing much more than is necessary. But I'm not sure about that. I'm telling my doctor I want to be more aggressive with my treatment. He says I'm in a healthy area now and don't need stronger treatment. He says, 'We're monitoring you very closely. If there's any major change, there'll be plenty of time to get you on a stronger treatment. We won't let you get sick.' But I think dropping this or that test or this or that drug is like needing a bodyguard twenty-four hours a day and then dropping it for an hour or so a day to save some money. Well, how do you know you won't be attacked during that hour? It's the same thing. If you don't monitor this particular blood test for six months or a year, you wouldn't know if it's dropping or not. I think that's why I get tested so much. The more information that you give them, the more they can discover, the better your chances of getting proper treatment. That's just the way I was brought up, having a lot of doctors in the family and having a lot of faith in medical science. To me, knowledge is the most important thing."

For Ron, diseases were like intruders and medical tests were like bodyguards. Ron didn't need to know what each of the lab tests meant. Except for making sure he had access to whatever was available, Ron trusted his physician to know what he was doing, just like he trusted his car to the mechanic. This rather mechanistic understanding of the body fit nicely into the structures that sustain medical consumption. But by accepting the dominant cultural model of health as his own, Ron experienced little of the conflict and discomfort apparent in many of the stories to come.

Ron was more positive about AZT and Western medicine than anyone I interviewed. For many, AZT brought up connotations of death or a futile last-ditch effort. Others decided they wanted AZT if they needed it, but took it without enthusiasm. Even Matthew, who insisted that his physician give it to him before his T cells were less than 500, didn't talk about it in the terms of hope that Ron did. However, Ron's belief in AZT was not fanatical either. When his doctor suggested that it would be better for him to wait, he accepted the advice, even as he attributed the drop in his T cells to the lack of aggressive intervention. Ron wasn't blindly uncritical of his "high-society" doctor, but he understood his doctor to be on the cutting edge rather than in the mainstream. This was important because the mainstream seemed to lead to death.

Some of those cutting-edge physicians and patients are now dead. Today the best research done on AZT suggests that it may have done more harm than good.[2] The Chinese herbal formula Resist may do as much good as AZT (and certainly less harm), but a person like Ron would never have taken the Chinese herb unless his Western physician had prescribed it. What was significant about Ron and James's new physicians was that they offered hope. They took chances. They treated their patients as they were treating themselves, within a shared system of knowledge and beliefs.

There were other cutting-edge physicians who never prescribed AZT, but they didn't just monitor blood work either. Like James and Ron's, these physicians were able to function as shamans or healers as well as scientists. What they offered was not simply the idea of hope, but a practice of hope. Cutting-edge physicians understood that to achieve a placebo effect is to achieve healing. This is true whether that effect is facilitated through AZT, Chinese herbs, or the physician's simple incantation "Everyone does not have to die from this." But none of this can work without a shared system of knowledge and beliefs.

▼▼▼

"Tell me about sex, drugs, and disco."

"HIV hurt my sex life for just a few weeks. That's one good thing I got from the counselor at the clinic. She told me this was going to happen and that I'd get over it. Sure enough, it did happen. I'm not monogamous, and it was several weeks before I dared to have sex with somebody. Even though I was practicing safe sex before, I didn't want to have sex at all. You know, you feel dirty, unclean, all that kind of stuff. Plus you're worried that somebody else might get you sick again. After I finally did have sex, it was fine. I've never had a problem since. It's like having an operation on your behind. The first time you take a bowel movement, it's horrible, and after that you have no problem."

"So what do you consider unsafe?"

"Well, I'm more of a sexual prude than a lot of people. I can get into a lot of game playing, but when it comes to exchanging bodily fluids, you know, shit and piss and all that kind of stuff never turned me on. In fact, I was always sort of prissy. It always turned me off. I'm not that big of a cocksucker either. I mean, it's fine, but I don't like them to cum in my mouth. Other people just love it, but I've never been big for that. If someone wants to take mine, that's fine, but I'm not a big recipient.

"The one unsafe thing that I used to do all the time was that I'd fuck and get fucked a lot. I cut that out almost entirely. It took me almost a year to be able to do it with rubbers. I didn't want to do it with rubbers, so I figured, if I'm not going to do it with rubbers, I'm not going to do it at all. Unsafe anal sex would be the only thing I would have liked to keep doing, which is probably what got me where I am now. As for the rest, AIDS got me off the hook. I don't have to seem like a prude anymore. Instead of saying, 'I don't want to or I'm not into it,' I can say, 'Well, we shouldn't do it.' So it was a good excuse.

"I actually know a lot of people who were not into anal sex. I had a roommate who always felt like he was an outsider because he didn't like fucking. He always had to make excuses. Safe sex was the greatest thing for him because he didn't have to make excuses anymore. There were certainly times when I had anal sex when I didn't want to. I just felt, well, okay, if they want to do it, let's do it and get it over with. When James and I got together, he didn't want me to get fucked, and he didn't particularly want me fucking people either. He didn't like anal sex because of VD and all that kind of stuff. He thought it was just too intimate. So I pretty much cut back on that eight years ago and did it very rarely.

"Drugs? I never was that big on drugs, but then I got big on drugs a few years back with the discos and all that stuff. Then I just loved it, but I always knew it was bad for me."

"What drugs?"

"Oh, anything! Like Ecstasy, crystal, and worse."

"What's worse than crystal? Heroin?"

"No. I've never done heroin. But I've done opium and I did dust [PCP] once. I hated that. I always knew drugs were bad for me, so I didn't like to do them too often, but I did like to do them once in a while for a party or special occasion."

"So in your drug heyday, about how often would you do a major drug? Once a week? Once a month?"

"Maybe once a month, but more like once every two to three months. When I did it, though , I did a lot. I mean, if I did it for a night, I didn't just do a little bit. I did a lot. I overdid it."

"What's the longest time you were ever awake on, say, crystal or coke?"

"Oh, only one night's sleep. I wouldn't go two nights without sleeping."

"So you didn't go on three-day binges?"

"No. Never. I had a job with responsibilities. I have a brain. I know that the stuff is bad for you. It can be fun for seven or eight hours, but after that it's going to be lousy. I didn't want to give up things like the gym and work. Of all the times I've done drugs, I never missed a day of work. It's like, if you're going to play on Saturday night, you'd better be real together by Monday morning. So once I did it, I'd be a pig with it. Then when AIDS came along, I still did it, even after I was positive, but I wasn't a pig. I might still do it every two or three months, but a much smaller dosage. In the last couple of months I've only taken a couple of hits off a joint, which I could care less about. I'm not that big on marijuana. In the last few months I have probably been clean longer than I've been since I was sixteen."

"What about alcohol?"

"I sometimes go weeks without drinking. Occasionally I'll have a beer or two on the weekend. Alcohol has never been big in my family. I'm not even a social drinker. I smoked for years, but if I smoke half a cigarette once every six months, that would be a lot. So smoking and drinking were things I did not cut back on when I found out that I was HIV positive. And I was only into drugs for about four or five years, from 1980 to 1985 or '86. Even then I didn't do them a lot. Every two or three months. Maybe on New Year's Eve or Halloween."

"So what drugs will you do for this New Year's?"

"Oh, I don't think I'm going to do any. That is not a promise, but I'm not even tempted. In fact, someone phoned me up who does it and offered me some stuff, and I said no. It's not a matter of trying to clean up my act. It's just that I'm sort of bored with it. Sometimes you outgrow things, and I think James and I are both starting to outgrow it. It's just not the turn-on anymore. Beyond the medical things, we don't like the way we feel after doing drugs, and we know we don't look pretty while we're doing it! And the late-night hours in the discos lately are getting boring, too. I think when the Saint closed in New York, that was the end of my disco days. I mean, I don't even like going to the I-Beam or Dreamland anymore. I used to get off on it. I used to love dancing. I'm not trying to sound like Polly Perfect."

"Oh, I know you're not Polly Perfect."

"I don't really do drugs on my own, but if I'm around certain friends, I do them. One of my friends from New York, a guy I used to run around with, is getting worse and worse into drugs—crack and everything. I look at him now and it's such a total turnoff that I don't want to be around him anymore.

"I do have a few friends here that I used to do drugs with who are HIV positive and have blood counts lower than mine. They don't want to do drugs anymore, but I would do drugs with them, if they wanted to. I like being around them, so if they wanted to go for long walks and knit sweaters, I'd probably want to do that with them. If they wanted to do drugs and have wild sex, I'd do that, too. I just like being with them. I'm sort of a follower that way, so if they're not doing drugs, I'm not doing drugs. Even drinking is the same. If my friend orders a Calistoga and I was going to have a beer, I'll just order a Calistoga. I'm sort of a copycat person. Not with everybody, just with certain people. So my act has sort of been cleaned up for me."

▼ ▼ ▼

Community exerted enormous influence throughout many of our lives, from sex, to drugs, to doctors. Sexual behaviors were at least partially constructed and modulated by our partners. Like Ron, many of us occasionally engaged in activities in which we had little interest, just because it was easier to go along than it was to refuse. Ron approached safe sex in a pragmatic manner and used it as an "excuse" so that he didn't have to be thought of as a prude anymore. When his lover wanted him to stop having anal sex with other people, he decreased that dramatically as well. If his buddies wanted to "do drugs and have wild sex," he would probably do them to stay connected. He'd also be happy knitting sweaters if that's what they wanted to do. High-risk behaviors in general were modulated by his friends more than they were by his own willpower or rational decision making.

In many ways Ron's approach to HIV was very holistic—reducing drug use, exercising, sleeping, staying connected with others, working together with his physician, being optimistic. However, the changes Ron made in his life were far more relational than they were ideological. Ron never called his approach holistic. In fact, activities like meditation and self-healing produced nothing but revulsion and guilt for him. Ron had a bit of holistic positive thinking in him. He liked to cheer people up. But Ron's positive thinking didn't function as a dogma or oppressive standard, not for himself or for anyone else.

Quiet Hope: Brian

I didn't know Brian nearly as well as I did Nathan, Matthew, and Ron. Brian worked in the travel industry and was a friend of Ron's. Ron actually told me that Brian wanted me to interview him as well, and I thought it made sense to talk with a few people I hadn't specifically selected. Brian wanted to come to my house for our talk. We sat in the living room and my eleven-foot Christmas tree made his face light up like a little kid's. The interview with Brian alerted me to the fact that I was concentrating on men who were very verbal, outgoing, and even somewhat aggressive. Brian was as quiet and introverted as the others were expressive and extroverted. He was quite aware that his concerns and approach to dealing with HIV were different from his friend Ron's, and he told a different kind of story.

▼ ▼ ▼

"Sometimes the four of us in the building talk about it—me, Ron, James, and Curtis. I don't really need to talk about HIV much. But I don't really like Ron's attitude about it. He's got the best numbers, but it's easier for me to talk with James—about anything actually. Ron is too obsessed; he gets on tangents about it. He's just far stronger, and his feelings about everything are harder. James and I take a softer attitude toward most things. We just do what we have to do, whereas Ron gets all hyped up and makes speeches about what we have to do. But that's the way he takes out the garbage. He's much more intense. It's not surprising that he's tremendously more successful at his work than James and I. She's a driven woman! If we're going to a movie and maybe have to wait five minutes for Curtis, James and I will be very easygoing, you know, pick up the paper or a magazine and read. But Ron is like a dog who has to pee. He's really very nice—all heart, you know, but he is not a relaxing presence. If you ever have a conversation with the two of them, Ron will dominate, and James and I would just as soon let him dominate."

We chatted about Ron and other mutual friends for a while before the conversation shifted to Brian's story.

"I have a woman friend who's a doctor in New York. It's really nice having a good friend who's a physician. She takes care of my medical stuff for me, and I bring back dolls for her children from around the world. That's our trade-off. When I thought I should be tested, she tested me. The test came back positive and that disturbed me, but it wasn't too overpowering at the time because I was expecting a positive result. Soon after that we decided to have the T cells done. So Shirley did the T cells, and they came back around 600 or so. I thought that was reasonable; that was okay at the time. It was really kind of casual. It was done in this way where I go in, she would do blood work, we'd have lunch, I'd see the kids. It wasn't as if I was sitting in a doctor's office waiting to have my T cells done and finding out I was positive. It was really comfortable. You know, here was this woman I'd known for ten, fifteen years, doing all this stuff. She was a physician who was good at her work and someone who I could really feel comfortable with, someone who really cared about me. Then the T cells came back at 180."

"All of a sudden?"

"Yeah. Like four months later, August of '89. I was back in New York for a couple of weeks and met Shirley at her office shortly after I arrived. A week later when I went over to see her and the kids, the results had come back. 180.

"And then I had to see my parents. They live in Ohio but were visiting in New York, so I had to see them. My dad really wanted me to take out something to do with life insurance or a twenty-year bond or something really long-term. They had made some investments that had worked okay for them and thought I should do it, too, but it would have entailed putting money away for twenty years or something. And here I had just found out my T cells were 180. It was really hard to think about a twenty-year anything. That was really the worst. That was really hard. I wish they hadn't been there."

"Did you tell them?"

"No. There was no reason to tell them. I had to get used to it before I could even discuss it with them. It never even occurred to me to tell them. I just hoped that if we started to argue that I wouldn't blurt it out. So, no, I wouldn't bring it up. They still don't know about all those tests. I think I told them I was positive, and it was never mentioned again. It was just an awkward weekend. I heard this news about the T-cell drop, and they were visiting on the same day. It was just really bad timing. I just wanted to get home and start dealing with the situation. After I returned from that layover in New York, I was able to start actively dealing with it, I guess.

"After seeing the count of 180, Shirley said she'd start AZT immediately if it was her. When I got back here, my San Francisco doctor said the same thing. I asked him, 'Should I be worried?'—and he answered, 'Do you want to be worried?' That's pretty much how I go through the day or the week about it. Sometimes it's on my mind all the time, and sometimes I don't think about it at all. A lot of people have perfectly healthy lives, taking AZT or dealing with it in other ways. At first it was strange having to take pills every three or four hours or whatever. But every time I thought, oh, this is kind of horrible, it became less horrible. Eventually, it all became part of the process. It was all right. The attitude I take is to be as relaxed as I can about this. I don't feel the need to run to the library to read up about all kinds of treatments. Everyone takes a different approach to it. I have to trust my doctor, and I have to trust myself to take good care of myself. Hopefully, that will be enough—because otherwise I think I could really upset myself a lot."

Taking AZT was not totally unproblematic for Brian, however. He did not have to deal with the efficacy issue or the poison issue. His trust in his physicians and in medicine relieved him of those potential conflicts. For Brian, it was neither being HIV positive nor having low T cells that reduced his worth as a potential boyfriend or lover. And whereas AZT was initially "horrible" for him, it no longer signified impending doom—except in one very special situation.

"Ed is my problem with this whole thing now. We were on our second date, about forty dates ago. Ed's beautiful, you know. He's just the best. But he doesn't feel he's at all good-looking. He's awkward with his body. He's so big. He really feels he got shafted, that he's not attractive at all. I couldn't quite understand what he was talking about, and then finally he said, 'There are things about me you just don't know.' So I asked, 'Do you want me to know?' Finally I dragged it out of him, and he said he was positive, and I said, 'So am I,' and we never brought it up again. It was never discussed. I know he goes to acupuncture."

"You've never discussed it again?"

"We've never discussed it again. I don't know why, and now I wish we had gone a little further into it sometimes. I really don't know the answer to this question. Should I tell Ed I'm on AZT? Do you think he has the right to know? It's an ethical, moral question, I guess. I just don't know whether I am comfortable telling him yet. I don't know if he has to know this yet. I have a feeling that the longer this goes on, the harder it's going to be to tell him. I went on AZT in August and then met Ed around Halloween. We haven't been apart a day since. A lot of people don't know I'm on AZT. I mean, good friends know I'm on AZT. It's hardly a secret. But he never asked, and I never asked him."

"Did you ever ask him what his T cells were?"

"I don't know what his T cells are."

"Does he know?"

"I have no idea. He lost a lover about five years ago to cancer. Then he spent the last year, from what I heard, traveling around the world trying to find some sort of cure. He said he could never, never deal with a lover dying again. There's a lot of pressure on me."

"You're not allowed to get sick or die?"

"No. This is really a tough one for me. I would not want Ed out of my life. I'm putting it off now because it's Christmas and I'm not going to tell him now. I don't know if I'm ever going to tell him. I asked my doctor about it, and he said, 'Well, you're certainly the millionth one who's come in with the same problem.' He thinks I should tell him. What would you do? Do you think I should tell him? I can imagine losing his lover was frightening for him. It's funny. I don't see myself as getting sick. I feel fine. I know lots of guys have said that before. But I don't know what I could tell him, if I should tell him, if he has a right to know, if I have an obligation to tell him."

"He may be on AZT, too."

"Yeah, he might. He might. I couldn't say why I don't think he is. I don't know. He could be. Who knows what his T cells are? There are lots of possibilities. I can only say that it wouldn't matter to me if he had 100 or 200 or 300 T cells. You know, we've never had anything but a lot of safe sex. It was never even discussed. It was always understood from the very start. So all that has been fine."

"Are you afraid that if you tell him he might go away?"

"Yes."

"Are you planning to wait until he's hooked first and then tell him?"

"He's hooked now. He asked me if I loved him yesterday. I was laughing and said, 'Oh God—I don't know.'"

"You said you didn't know?"

"I didn't know if he was serious about it. You know, Richard, every ten years when someone tells me they love me—"

He chuckled softly.

"I don't have a lot of experience with this kind of thing, and it came out of, out of the blue. It also has to do a lot with my self-image. I mean, I look at him and I think he's the greatest gift. You know, he's my best Christmas present. He's like the best toy I ever had. I don't want anything to mess that up right now. I'm really thankful for him. Maybe it's the season, you know, the holiday season and all. I'm not really a challenging kind of guy. I don't probe a lot. It doesn't matter to me. I'm certainly happy with him. I don't know. If he was on AZT, who am I to think anything of it? We could sit and take our pills together, I guess. That would be one thing, but, uh—"

"Well, you're so in love, you're just caught."

"Oh, puke, right? Isn't that just terrible? Am I misting? Well, you know I've wanted a boyfriend for a long time, since I've moved here."

"It's the nurse in me, I guess. I would never want to know somebody's T cells for the basis of whether I wanted to be their lover or not. But I would always want to know their T cells so we could talk about what they should do, to give them my advice and to get theirs. It sounds like you're sort of relying on your doctor to advise you and his doctor to advise him. Is that right?"

"Yeah. I guess that's about right. I trust his judgment totally. I just think he's really smart and probably capable of taking care of his business. I don't know; this is really, really personal. Maybe we're not ready to go into it yet."

▼▼▼

Even though Brian lived in a building with three other HIV-positive friends, even though he lived in a community that overtly dealt with the virus on a daily basis, Brian seemed somewhat isolated in relation to HIV. He "thinks" he mentioned being HIV positive to his parents, but it was never mentioned again. Brian had a quiet approach to things in general, but sometimes he seemed so quiet that he barely gave expression to his hopes or fears. Yet I didn't feel that his feelings were stuck or that he needed counseling.

Personally, I couldn't imagine not talking about T cells with a boyfriend or lover. But I sometimes forgot that I was a nurse and that these issues were somewhat overdetermined for me. People in my community were coping with HIV in very different ways. The issue was too "personal" to discuss with a boyfriend. Brian was in a relationship where not talking about certain issues was normative, and he was reluctant to let health concerns dominate how that relationship developed.

Brian didn't need to discuss HIV with his friends in his building. For Brian, HIV was something to discuss with medical personnel. He trusted doctors to make decisions about HIV, both for himself and for his boyfriend. He even asked his doctor for advice about what he should disclose to his boyfriend, something the doctor had been asked a million times. But Brian hadn't resolved all of these issues with his doctor, which may have been part of why he wanted to talk with me.

"We had a really interesting problem last week. Ed just bought a building, and he has to rent out the in-law apartment to cover the mortgage. A very nice guy came by, and Ed found out he had 22 T cells. Then Ed decided not to rent to him because he was just afraid that this guy could get sick, and Ed wouldn't be able to turn him out on the street because he just couldn't do that. But then he wouldn't be able to cover the mortgage. He felt really bad because if we turn against each other, if we turn each other down, who's going to help us out? He felt this was really bad. He had a real hard time with it. The guy was fine. The guy had a good job. I asked him, 'Well, what would happen if this guy had a million T cells and lost his job and couldn't afford the rent? You'd be in the same kind of position.' But Ed said if he wasn't sick he could ask him to leave and it would be a lot easier.

"These are the kinds of things that are on my mind these days. I feel good; I take care of myself as well as I can. But suddenly I feel I have somebody else to consider who I suspect is going to be around a long time in my life."

Brian understood the importance of social support in our community. Whereas Brian was reluctant to tell Ed about being on AZT, he did not feel alienated from his community in general, but his community was nonetheless experiencing some alienation within itself. Whether to disclose one's antibody status, T-cell counts, or prescription drugs like AZT to a new lover or whether to rent an apartment to someone with low T cells was not always an easy decision.

At the same time, the community still had a sense of idealism, expressed through an almost mythic allegiance toward those who had died. The Quilt, memorial groves, and AIDS literature and art signified loves and friendships sustained long after death. Those for whom we grieved became heroes who showed us what remained possible in the midst of suffering and death. Although the community inevitably experienced some continued alienation within itself, it also responded to many of the moral quandaries and crises besetting it. AIDS organizations started addressing housing issues, and the AIDS Emergency Fund paid the rent for many who might otherwise lose their homes or create financial hardship for their HIV-positive landlords. Brian had a quiet trust in his physicians, but the strength and comfort he needed to face illness and death he found in his community.

▼ ▼ ▼

"I know so many people who've passed away, and they were great guys. They were just real models, guys who had huge careers or huge personalities, or they had something really special about them. And I think, having seen all these guys go before me, I'd be in good company if something happened to me."

"So they had some sort of belief about life after death or—"

"Yeah, but I'm not clear on it. I have a feeling that something else is going on. I don't know exactly what's out there. I don't think I'm going to go to heaven and see all these old friends and we're going to, you know, hang out. But I figure there's some sort of transformation that's going to happen. I just don't know what. It almost doesn't even matter. I don't have to know. I can't see myself as just bones in a ditch. It doesn't seem like that's it either. But having seen all these guys go off before me really helped in some ways. I mean, these guys were heroes."

"How were they heroes?"

"The dignity and the class that they showed when they were sick enables me never to be afraid. These guys were, you know, such examples. I'd be proud to be with these guys in that way, to learn something from them. They were my, some of my favorite people. It's almost like I couldn't let them down."

"I know what you mean."

"I think I would have been a horrible example if something had happened to me earlier on, but now it's a lot easier. Being here in San Francisco certainly makes it easier. The idea that I would have Ron, James. Maybe Ed. It's hard to say what would happen. I don't think about it a lot. I just don't. What would happen if I got really, really ill? It crosses my mind. But since I don't know what would happen, having these guys around would make it better. Better than anything. Better than any other situation I could possibly envision.

| 6 |

During the 1950s and 1960s the mere presence of a gay bar gave license for police raids and arrests of patrons who might be seen cross-dressed, dancing, or holding hands. In 1969 a group of drag queens in New York had enough. The freedom to enjoy cocktails at the Stonewall bar became their "line in the sand,"[1] and once that line was firmly drawn, the butch boys came out as well. Over the next few years several variations on "gay macho" became visible in our community, and the Boys in the Band, miserable and bitter by comparison, were joined by a new generation of sugarcoated hedonists typified by the Village People.

In San Francisco the typical "Castro clone" was fashioned to both look and perform like a perpetual hard-on: hiking boots, tight 501 Levi's, long-sleeved flannels or short-sleeved Lacoste shirts; short hair, mustaches. No frills. Many wore workman keys on the right or left to indicate top or bottom. Full black leather was another option. Even drag queens sported mustaches and beards as gender-fuck became both a political statement and an art form. We celebrated our sexuality and our masculinity, and for many of us it was the first time in our lives.

We had bars for leathermen, bars for sweater queens, bars for young boys, for drag queens, for video buffs, for hustlers and their tricks, and for people who just wanted to drink or dance. Even the baths were specialized. There were baths for gym boys, for the S&M crowd, for fist-fuckers, and a giant bathhouse open twenty-four hours a day, seven days a week, for people who were just horny.

We met gay men everywhere in our new village, not just in bars, discos, and bathhouses, but on the street, in the grocery store, on the bus, at the beach—even at the VD clinic. Cruising never stopped in the San Francisco that Armisted Maupin captured in his classic *Tales of the City*. For many of my friends, a typical year in the decade preceding AIDS included from two hundred to three hundred different sexual partners. Do that over a decade or so and it's not hard to accumulate the somewhat astonishing number of two to three thousand partners. Sex was the primary means through which many gay men sought, met, and related to each other during the 1970s and early 1980s. Eric and I were no exception. Almost all our friendships started out sexually. We even joked that it was best to get the sexual tension out of the way so that friendship might have a chance.

We referred to our sexual liaisons as "tricks," "fuck-buddies," "boyfriends," and "lovers." The desire for monogamy or some sort of ongoing relationship on the part of one or both partners produced the boyfriend category—guys who were "dating" or "seeing" each other. "Lover" was used for our equivalent of a heterosexual marriage. Of course, it wasn't equivalent entirely. Parental approval was rarely an issue in those days, although some of us did distinguish between those you could and could not take home to meet the folks.

Liberal heterosexuals frequently misinterpreted the meaning of "lover" in the gay community. A colleague once complained that a gay student kept referring to his lover during an evaluation conference. Trying to show support, I responded, "If a student talked about her husband during an evaluation conference, I'd be annoyed as well."

"No," she continued. "He was talking about his lover, not his partner. He was shoving his sex life in my face."

"He was inappropriate, but he wasn't shoving his sex life in your face," I explained. "Lovers are the gay equivalent for spouses."

"It's not the same," she insisted. "Sex isn't necessarily a part of marriage. Lovers are sexual."

It took some time to convince her that we did indeed use the term *lover* for spouse. She couldn't understand why we would use such an illicit word for our permanent relationships, no doubt thinking of the connotations associated with the nineteenth-century use of the term. Alas, sex between gay "lovers" disappears as often as it does among heterosexual married couples. However, many of our marriages were "open," and tricks, fuck-buddies, or the boyfriend-on-the-side played the equivalent of the illicit heterosexual "lover."

The man we picked up in a bar, at the supermarket, or off the street was a "trick." A meal or movie together was not sufficient to move out of the trick category, but a trick could move to fuck-buddy, boyfriend, or lover over time. The fuck-buddy category was highly valued among people like Eric and me. Fuck-buddies were people who could be depended on for good, no-strings-attached sex, people whose names we knew and whose phone numbers were already in the black book. Fuck-buddies might share romantic feelings, friendship, or even love, but marriage was never the goal. Three or four good fuck-buddies was heaven.

For most of us, drugs were an integral part of the party. Aside from the pleasures they brought, marijuana and other drugs often signified a common link between gay people and the larger, mostly heterosexual counterculture. When the Kennedy assassinations, Vietnam, and Richard Nixon annihilated the collective fantasy of *Father Knows Best*, a wide generation gap was born in the United States. Even though "turn on, tune in, drop out" quickly degenerated into mindless sensuality, the movement began as a moral response to what was, for many, an amoral establishment.

To this gay hippie, the pot smoking and occasional psychedelic "tripping" among gay men in the early 1970s seemed mostly harmless. Many of us never even counted marijuana as a drug. It was simply kept in a canister next to the flour and sugar. When poppers came on the scene, they did not seem like drugs either. They weren't even illegal. I used to wear a small metal container on a leather thong around my neck. That way I could offer a sexual or dance partner a "hit" wherever and whenever it might seem appropriate. I didn't even like poppers very much. They were part of the "look," a kind of fashion statement.

During the late 1970s and early 1980s this scene changed dramatically. In San Francisco the proliferation of bathhouses and the all-night megadisco parties created a perfect medium for drugs of all kinds, especially speed and cocaine. A few people even started shooting them. My own attitudes toward drugs took a sharp turn the day some guy talked me into smoking a Quaalude. "'Ludes come on stronger when you smoke 'em," he insisted. I had always thought the beauty of Quaaludes was their subtlety. Drugs were no longer a social statement, a protest, or even simple hedonism. It all stopped making sense. People were indiscriminately mixing so many drugs together that they couldn't possibly experience the particular high that any of them had to offer. This was even true for the new designer drugs, such as "MDA," drugs that were carefully balanced to make one simultaneously energized and relaxed, high enough to fly and focused enough to fuck.

By the late 1980s we were shoving both crystal methamphetamine and a large-animal tranquilizer we called "K" up our noses, not just at the baths, but at white parties, black parties, and street fairs. For a while it seemed as if every celebration would find some muscle number stuck in a "K-hole," stopped dead in his tracks, like a deer staring into headlights. Many of us walked a very fine line between simple abuses and serious addiction. We didn't skimp on the alcohol either. Sex, drugs, and alcohol defined the venues where we met. Thus, when AIDS hit the gay community, it was far more than a medical crisis. AIDS threatened a whole way of life, an entire subculture. Diseases and their accompanying medical tests and treatments came to tower over the landscape of our newly liberated lives, often turning a garden of earthly delights into a little shop of horrors.

I'm not sure whether these indulgences resulted from a collective unconscious terror of our nuclear age, our alienation from a homophobic society, self-hatred, or a combination of factors. In one way or another many people with HIV/AIDS lived at the extreme margins of the culture, either as gay men, drug users, or both. Consequently, very few AIDS researchers could even fathom how a man might have more than two thousand sexual partners and still hold a job. Very few understood the attraction of speed sex or the rush from crack cocaine or a hit of poppers during orgasm. Likewise, many researchers and clinicians steeped in modern medical understandings found it difficult to comprehend why some men were reluctant to monitor T cells or take antivirals.[2] Health professionals would eventually come to understand the virus better than they would those who lived with it.

During the late 1980s many gay men were as serious about sex and partying as some of our heterosexual counterparts were about sports. Some still are. Eric has been one of our star sexual athletes, excelling in the singles competitions. Jason used to cheer on the team by organizing our celebrations, hosting our parties, and bringing us all together. Eric's and Jason's understanding of HIV and AIDS was very different from the preceding stories. Eric insisted that the destruction of the gay subculture was killing more gay men than the virus. Eric worked on deconstructing the political/medical understanding of AIDS and thought that its solution was a radical realignment of social power. Jason thought that the expectation of death and disease was creating its own inevitability, that negative thinking was the most dangerous aspect of HIV. Jason tried hard to keep negative psychological metaphors out of his mind, but that required a radical reconstruction of his own nature. Both stories provide important alternative scenarios for coming to terms with HIV.

The Heresy of Social Science: Eric

Eric was a graduate student and a real enigma to me. We'd spent considerable time sharpening ideas as academic sparring partners. When we weren't discussing sex or men, we usually argued about the structure, distribution, and function of contemporary power. We both admired Michel Foucault and were particularly critical of the health "sciences." But one thing I simply could not fathom was his repeated assertion that he did not "believe" in T cells. Whenever we talked about T cells or AZT, he would insist that submitting to either amounted to "selling out" to the medical establishment.

I arrived at Eric's house at 10:30 A.M. Although we had spoken on the phone two hours earlier, he answered the door in a bathrobe. We were good friends. He was talking on the phone with tonight's "date." I was somewhat surprised when Eric asked the guy what his T cells were, and I jokingly interrupted to say, "You can't ask those questions. You don't believe in T cells. Those are my questions." After hanging up the phone, he disappeared into the shower. "How stupid!" he hollered from the bathroom. "This guy is taking AZT."

We went for breakfast and then to my house for our interview. When I asked Eric when he first thought about protecting himself sexually, he invoked an ex-lover to answer my question.

"Well, it depends what you mean by protecting. I think I'm a product of the time in that I was very driven to have sex. I learned very quickly, and sex developed into a medium for communication. When I was eighteen, I was living in Watsonville with a boyfriend, Lonnie. He never wanted me to go up to San Francisco because whenever I came back, he thought I was physically or emotionally traumatized. Lonnie thought that I had trouble saying no. We had long conversations on how to say no and how to be more protective of my body and of my person.

He even thought I had a self-destructive streak that I expressed through sex."

"Which a lot of us do. It was almost part and parcel of the sexual experience, part of the liberation."

"True. But back then gay men were objectifying each other in the most extreme ways. Men have a tendency to objectify people anyway, and in the gay community there were no barriers and no restraints on those tendencies. People were nasty. They didn't think of the other person as a person. They were basically disregardful."

"Is that really how you would characterize gay sex in the '70s and early '80s?"

"Lots of things were going on, but that was definitely a component. People expressed an anger toward each other and toward themselves, especially in the way cruising happened, the attitude people had, the way people took sexual cruising as an insult."

"What? People took cruising as an insult?"

"Sure. A lot of times. People reacted to someone showing interest, like, 'Ugh, how dare you!'"

"Oh, that, 'I'm so much prettier than you; how could you think for a minute that I would be interested in you?' That sort of thing?"

"Yeah. It was ruthless. I think we treated each other badly, very badly. I'm convinced that that's partly why AIDS happened. We were abusing each other and ourselves. I think that created the pathways for disease to spread. That was the opening. The gay community was very sexual. I even wrote about it at the time. I called it sexual fascism, the oppressive and pervasive imperative to have sex all the time. That was the atmosphere. That was the medium in which everything was decided and expressed. All your worth was based on sex and based on looks, and it was really oppressive. I actually left San Francisco because of it. Around '80, '81, I was getting kind of disenchanted with it and wanted to leave. So I went to New York."

We both started laughing at the notion of escaping sexual fascism by moving from San Francisco to New York. "Completely different!" I said sarcastically.

"Well, there was also this obligatory happiness in San Francisco. You had to be happy all the time. You couldn't be a naysayer. At the time both Kyle [his best friend] and I were sort of having trouble fitting in and being comfortable with what was going on. We were getting a lot of shit for it. We couldn't just go to the all-night discos. We couldn't just go to the bathhouses. We just weren't at ease. I actually never had much trouble. When we went to the Jaguar [a bookstore/sex club], there was this big, tall, very sexy guy who I would always interact with. But Kyle would never have fun. Kyle would never connect. I understood what he was talking about because I had some of those feelings, too. It just never prevented me from connecting, but I was still kind of uneasy about everything. I remember walking out of there and down Eighteenth Street toward Castro Street with Kyle shaking his head going, 'It's wrong. Something's up. This isn't going to work out.' He broke his Jaguar card in half and said, 'Eric, something's up. This whole thing is going to come crashing down.' People would comment on how depressed we were, and we thought at some point they're all going to get unhappy like us. And later we thought we were right.

"When I went to New York, I drove across the country and did what I still really like to do—which is to fuck my way across the country. In Chicago I met this guy at the Gold Coast. We went back to his place and had a great time. He was really fun, and he fucked me. This was back in '81, and people were still fucking to the point of cumming. The whole idea of condoms wasn't there yet. But you want to know something odd? Kyle and I figured that it had to be anal intercourse around '81/'82. We just figured it out based on what was going on and who got it and who didn't and how widespread it was and wasn't. We decided that it had to be something as specific as that."

Since Eric had figured out that AIDS was related to anal sex around 1981–1982, I wondered what he thought about Larry Kramer's work. Kramer had been the leading voice against promiscuous sex from within the gay community. Eric had read it but didn't buy it:

"I thought Kramer was ridiculous and hysterical. I knew for my own self that there was no way I was going to stop having sex. AIDS wasn't even putting a dent into my sex life—even to the point of protective-ness. Yet these people were out and out saying, 'Don't have any sex,' or 'We have got to change everything.' I was becoming worried that the social ramifications of HIV were becoming worse than the physical ones, worse than the medical ones.

"Obviously we have a biological problem here, but this hysteria and this rejection—this wholesale rejection of gay culture, and even of gay sexuality, is compounding the problem immeasurably. People have forgotten that the gay community was aware of what was going on. In fact, at the end of '79 there was a manifesto type of thing in the *New York Native*—ten areas to deal with in the gay community. We were reaching a maturity on our own—without AIDS. We were reappraising our sexuality and our lifestyle in a very sober, serious way—in a constructive way.

"But then what happened? Instead of critically and constructively talking about gay life, Larry Kramer and the rest of them got hysterical about it. Instead of fixing it, instead of dealing with it, instead of going through all these problems, they were going to freeze them at that unresolved, unbalanced, horrible stage. On top of it all, they dumped all this guilt, all this recrimination, all this rejection of gay pride, the gay body, and gay sexuality. I thought that was going to hopelessly confound the situation, and I thought it was very dangerous. It very much fueled the epidemic and caused the collapse of the gay lifestyle in the major urban areas like New York and San Francisco. It ruined the way everyone lived without providing an alternative. On top of that, it made us completely vulnerable to the negative imaging and labeling powers of the AIDS construct and made us defenseless against the heterosexual onslaught. I personally believe that if AIDS had never been invented and defined the way it was, the epidemic would have been much smaller, much, much smaller."

"What do you mean by heterosexual onslaught. What's that got to do with the construction of AIDS?"

"I think that gay men were becoming very anxious about having moved far away from the rest of society. They wanted both to be gay and to be part of society, and it was impossible to be openly gay in an anti-gay society. You couldn't have full membership in the gay community and full membership in straight society. There had to be some sort of adjustment. Personally, I think there was a time when two value systems had matured to the point that they were in total competition. One had to give, and AIDS was used to get rid of the gay reality, basically."

The visible gay culture that emerged in the 1970s was in large measure based on a promiscuous hypersexuality. Many gay men were hypersexual for some easy-to-identify reasons: a homophobic culture, an alienated adolescence, the sexual revolution, the rejection of monogamy as a heterosexual value, the absence of a restraining and domesticating female energy, and for some, gay meccas or ghettos that allowed for the release of pent-up sexual and affectionate feelings. When AIDS threatened this hypersexuality, the whole gay subculture reverberated with the double whammy. Friends and lovers were dropping dead, and our newly constructed, newly liberated lives were turned upside down. Our whole orientation to sexual interaction with our own kind, always precarious because of the distrust and disgust it produced in the dominant culture, started becoming more visible, from Stonewall in New York to Gay Pride in San Francisco. But the hypersexual identity that emerged was fragile—politically, psychologically, and biologically.

Rather than a courageous act to save lives, Kramer's antipromiscuity position, as Eric saw it, was a myopic attempt to control bodies and feelings with rational social management. Eric thought that the public health and medical constructions of AIDS destroyed both our culture and our identity and in so doing ultimately took more lives than the virus. But it wasn't clear to me that the gay culture had really disappeared, even in Eric's very specific sexual sense. Eric didn't stop having sex—lots of the same kind of sex he had had before. And after hearing how horrible we had been to each other, how we had all objectified each other sexually, I wondered what of our gay culture Eric thought needed preserving. Yet Eric insisted that, while oppressive, our sexuality was also positive.

▼▼▼

"There was a sense of community that was glued together through sex, which I think was fine. There was just a sheer enjoyment of sex. Sex became a folk art, and people were busy practicing. It's like we were employing homophobic tendencies to break down our homophobic selves—to break down the man in us, to create a new gay individual, on a personal level and on a community level. Sex does have a masochistic aspect that is completely valid and unavoidable, though I think it reached a threshold that ultimately produced ill health.[3]

"There were two sides to it. The good side was the creation of a gay community and a gay personality. The bad side was the unhygienic and biologically destructive situation that followed. And we weren't very nurturing. In an all-male society the worth of a male is diminished. In an all-male society the worst of male values, the worst of the male personality, came out. We were very destructive and abusive. We used and exploited each other. We were not very nurturing or caring or loving at all, but all this had the effect of destroying the male ego and the male personality. It tended to break down the self and allow for a new self to be built."

"When was there a shift for you in any of that personally?"

"Well, who knows, if ever. I'm still pretty abusive and exploitative."

Several men in my research spoke of their selves being broken down and reconstructed through sex. This reconstruction of the self through sex often included the violation of both social and biological norms. Most men in this study spoke of this process in very positive terms and bemoaned the fact that it was nearly impossible to let go of the self in the age of AIDS. However, I'm not sure that the extent to which we were "used and exploited" by each other necessarily destroyed our male egos and male personalities. A culture of use and exploitation can reform or reinforce abusive tendencies. Indeed, it can do both.

Eric's interest in the emerging gay self was not just because of his investment in sexual freedom. Eric was concerned with our social relationships and wanted to sustain a discourse of morality and responsibility as well. Yet he never set himself up as an example for others to follow. When Eric said he was still abusive and exploitative, he was not just being modest. His ideology of gay male sexuality was nonobjectifying, nurturing, and caring, but the fact that his own behavior did not conform to this ideology was not problematic for him. Rather, it stood as evidence that another ideology was needed.

When Eric eventually moved from San Francisco to New York, his experience with sexual fascism was not replaced by a "life-affirming" gay sexuality. In the past Eric and I had talked about the differences between whores and sluts in the gay world (whores have sex for money; sluts do it for fun). We were both identified with the latter, but for the first time Eric revealed that in New York he had been a bit of both.

"I was beginning to date the very attractive, A-gay type in New York. It was real clear that I was having no trouble entering into those circles. I went out with a guy named Devon who was incredibly good-looking and who had a house on Fire Island and was known as being one of the stars of the A-gay track. I was dating the owner of the Chasm—both he and his lover. And I was living with an ABC executive on West Fourteenth Street. I mean it was just real clear that I had no trouble doing it. Devon and I even talked about it. He told me, 'You're smart and you're sexy. You're funny and you're different. You could be a professional at this stuff [as in a model/whore] if you liked,' and that confused me. Because, on the one hand, I was getting all that sexual attention, and on the other hand, sex was really dangerous.

"I was working in a bar, the Pigskin. It was a pretty sleazy bar, and I was getting gradually more and more uptight. I started wearing more and more clothes, and baggier and baggier clothes, and getting more and more nervous and resentful of the attention. Then the manager realized what was going on. He put a Quaalude on the bar in front of me and walked away and came back with a shot of something and said, 'Lookit, you just don't have the right attitude you're just not with us. Take this and you'll have more fun here.' Which I did. That worked for a couple of weeks, but I was unhappy.

"Then I sort of traded on the sex stuff more than I had been. I got paid more directly. Just to see what that was like. But the one time I did it I fell apart the next day. Absolutely fell apart. And it wasn't so much that I fell apart because I thought, oh my God, I did something like that. It was that I didn't feel in control of it. I felt that my whole world was being based on my ability to project a sexual energy and to weave sexual spells and that everyone's interest and desire for me was conditionally based on my ability to maintain the magic. It all meant that I was basically all alone. The sex was suspect anyway, because of AIDS, and dangerous. I just sort of fell apart, and it was all about issues of self-worth and drugs. It got very confusing for a poor little twenty-one-year-old to deal with.

"I was also dating Nick, this guy who was one of the New York stars. Even John-Claude, my ex-lover from the River, knew about him and said, 'Oh, you were going out with Nick! Oh my God.' I didn't want to go out with Nick, and yet I didn't know how to say no because he was, you know, such a catch, supposedly. I remember being on these dates and calling Lonnie, just in tears, saying how I wanted to go home, how this guy was killing me, and I just couldn't say no. And Lonnie would say, 'Walk over to him. Say you have to go home. Come back here. Hang up the phone.' After a month or two of that I finally left New York.

"But first there was this whole transitional period where I was fucking with this one guy, who I really liked, who worked at ABC in the publishing department. He was very cultured, and he really liked me—and in a much nicer way than these other people did. He was about ten years older. He had me read Henry James and told me things like, 'Now you are in New York, and I can see that it is kind of rough, but you can do it. There are just three things that you have to maintain, and that's food, shelter, and clothing. And as long as you keep those three at a certain level, you'll be all right.' And we would fuck, and we would fuck to the point of cumming inside. I didn't really fuck him. I really liked him physically, and I really liked my interactions with him. But every time we fucked I would go running into the bathroom to discharge it as fast as I could and look and look and look and examine it to see if there was any blood. If I'd been fucked without causing any blood, I'd be relieved. If there was blood, I would agonize and want to cry and sort of slap myself to get it back together and go back out to the bedroom."

"How do you account for still getting fucked without condoms after having decided that the behavior was linked to AIDS?"

"It just goes to show how obligatory sex was at the time, how absolutely essential it was to have sex. There is still a strong, forceful imperative to have sex. Back then it was truly oppressive."

"Wait a minute. You left San Francisco because of an oppressive social force that was driving everyone to fascist sex. Then you fucked your way across the country. Was there any individual component to your sexuality, or was it entirely socially constructed?"

"Well, yes, there was an individual part of it. But I also think that California was extreme. There were reasons why San Francisco developed the way it did. Men are very sexual anyway, and for gay men there were no restraints because they were doing it with other men. And gay men were hypersexual for other reasons. They had to prove their masculinity, and they didn't have access to the nonsexual ways of doing it that straight men did, like being a father, being a boss, and being a man in other traditional respects. In addition, California is a land of very recent immigrants who have very few ties to their pasts, to religion, to ethnicity, to ethnic community, and even to family. So friends, peers, and sexuality become more important because of the lack of these other factors that build up a personality. On top of that, California is late consumer capitalism par excellence. It is probably more impacted by advertising and the media than anywhere else. I was a product of all those: being a

Californian, being in San Francisco, being gay. It made me very sexual."

"You seem to have an intellectual perspective on yourself as a socially determined being. I'm interested in whether—either due to emotional things or spiritual things or experiential things—you ever separated yourself out. In terms of deciding to practice safe sex or protecting yourself, did you ever distinguish or separate yourself out in any way from the socially determined self? Did anything like that ever happen to you?"

"Well, I can do that, but we have to back up a little bit. In '80 or '81 I was still working on these ideas. I'd already written several papers, and I had really thought about this stuff. When I went to Chicago, I fucked with this guy and then later moved to New York. Remember the first *Time* article on AIDS? Well, the guy's picture was in it as one of the first people to come down with AIDS. I just gasped! It was shocking! It turned out he was the director of the Sherman theater and was very prominent in the Chicago gay community. Anyway, it was very upsetting. It made me very worried—made me feel exposed, contaminated, affected, all those things.

"It was also kind of confusing. I kept a record of my—you know—dates. I had an engagement calendar that I wrote everything down in, and if you look at my first couple months in New York, there was nearly a different person every single night. I really enjoyed it, but it also made me feel crazy because you feel kind of eaten up and torn apart and used and stuff. Then on top of that, knowing that you may have a life-threatening disease that you don't quite understand—it's terrifying. I was only twenty-one. It was all kind of confusing. I got very worried. I actually kind of fell apart emotionally, and I think that was all part of it."

After a relentless effort to get Eric to move from social commentary to his own story, he finally found a way back to himself by way of an article in *Time*! Eric seemed to understand himself as a socially constructed being who became individuated through sex. As a product of social forces, as a member of a culture undergoing a sexual revolution, as a Californian, he had to have a different person almost every night. And sex, socially and biologically constructed both to threaten and to affirm our physical health and our gay identity, was necessarily enjoyable and disturbing.

Whereas many academics think that people are at least partially socially constructed, almost all of Eric's self-understanding is expressed in these terms. Without the sexual culture, Eric almost didn't exist as an individual at all. The only time in our conversation that he consistently used the first-person voice was when he was relating sexual experiences. Even Eric's story about taking the HIV test was organized around the assault on his sexual system rather than around medical decisions or issues related to mortality.

▼ ▼ ▼

"At the end of '85 I got tested, and it came out positive. It was weird. It was definitely weird for me. That was probably the most destructive period of my sex life—even more than the early '80s. Suddenly, I didn't know when or how to talk to people. That was the first time my sexual behavior, my system, my approach, my strategy got threatened and dysfunctional. I still had sex, and I still wanted to have sex because that was my mode, my way of meeting people and stuff. Yet I was confused and didn't know what I should say or what I shouldn't say or if I could say it. I kind of didn't believe in it all, but then again I wasn't quite sure. So I would get paralyzed during sex.

"I didn't want to tell people I was positive because I hated the idea of being contaminated. At the same time, I felt that I should tell them. So it would bug me the whole time if I didn't tell them. I was also trying to figure out what everybody else's assumptions were: whether they were going under the assumption that people were negative unless you said something or whether they were going under the assumption that everyone was positive unless you said something; whether it was the positive person's responsibility to tell; whether it was the negative person's responsibility to ask; whether people prefer just not to know and if they did know, they were annoyed because you ruined the whole thing and interjected a note of death and gloom and doom into a sex-positive, life-enhancing situation. I was dealing with all those things, and I couldn't quite get a grip on it.

"Around that time I was really coming into my own in the sense that I found that I could get people who I really liked—really, really liked—if I wanted them. I really wanted this one guy that I thought was just gorgeous, absolutely the sexiest person ever. I kind of flirted, and he responded, and I thought, wow, this is neat. And it was literally a couple of weeks or a couple of days after I got tested, and the sex fell apart. Absolutely. I got really nervous and anxious and wasn't enjoying it. I finally told him in the middle of it. We'd been doing it for about an hour, and I was getting more and more uncomfortable, and finally I said, 'Look, I really have to tell you something.' And he just sort of stopped and said, 'I've been around the block, and you've been around the block. Don't worry about it.' But I never quite recovered and never really got back into the swing of it. It was really upsetting, and it definitely stopped the momentum for both of us. It kind of made him sad. Then he wanted to date again and wanted me to fuck him. I found that absolutely impossible, and it wasn't about the rubber. By then I was a little bit unbalanced with all my attitudes and all my fears and my desires. It was because he kept using Lube out of a container.[4] And this was '85, and in '82–'83 I had a horrible case of amoebas, and I was petrified that he kept using this Lube. So finally I told him that I couldn't use that Lube. He just thought that was too medicalized. I had totally disconnected him from the sex and desexualized the situation. I even thought I was crazy at the time."

Eric recounted this incident, four or five years after it had happened, as the most destructive of his sex life—even more destructive than the experiences he described in New York. A couple of awkward moments in an otherwise flawless record as one of our most accomplished sexual athletes—a single loss of sexual momentum was remembered as the most destructive force ever to penetrate his sexual system. It didn't seem to matter that he "got the girl" and eventually became lovers with the guy. Microorganisms and the stuff they grew in, together with the people and systems charged with fighting those microorganisms, had all invaded and disrupted Eric's sexual relationships. Because sexual relationships formed the basis for Eric's identity as a gay man, this disruption was devastating for him, as it was for many others in the community.

"For me the enemy has never been just the AIDS virus at all. The enemy has always been the medicalization process that has been more lethal than the virus itself—the whole loss of gay culture and the reinstitution of an antigay, medicalized, pseudoheterosexual culture. That scientists, politicians, and physicians have articulated this AIDS concept makes me right off the bat suspicious. I just know that institutionally it's going to have an antigay bias to it—both institutionally and ideologically. Second, I don't believe in the medical model in the sense that you focus solely on the biological model.

"You have got to remember in '85, '86—on the flimsiest statistical stuff, the flimsiest studies, when the epidemic was at its height in the sense of its chargedness, when the imaging powers were the most powerful—they manufactured the most lethal ideas and conceptions by writing right and left that everybody was going to die, that there was no hope, don't have sex at all—on the flimsiest of stuff. The studies were small, the statistics were worst-case scenarios, and they gleefully would say in the *New York Times* and other authoritative places how everybody who was positive was going to die. Now they're reevaluating it. Now they're saying, 'Gosh, that isn't how it is going to happen,' and that's buried on the tenth page. When they were telling everybody they were going to die, it was front-page news, headline stuff. I just felt the *Times* was irresponsible. Their wish for gay men to die was almost conscious.

"It wasn't just that we got infected with the virus. All this self-loathing and the destruction of gay culture made it impossible to live life in a normal, satisfactory, and sustaining way. Anthropology is really clear about this. There are a lot of studies of what is called boning—how people can be convinced to die, or compelled to die, from no apparent biological basis. But they are treated as if they are going to die, their relationships are cut off, they enter into a death role, and lo and behold they die within a week or two or within a month.

"So here you are, a gay man who has been told all his life that he is bad. You have developed this system to counter it; this ideology to counter it—gay liberation, all the other gay pride stuff, plus hypersex. You are already in a weakened state because you live in a homophobic society and physically because of the successive wave of diseases.[5] But you have an ideology that counters it, and suddenly that ideology is stripped away from you. In fact, you hear that it was wrong in the first place, which activates the homophobia that is at the basis of your personality. You no longer have access to all the ways of living that legitimized and gave you sustenance. Bad as they were, you no longer had any of that. You can't fuck, you can't do anything, but you still have those desires, so you're torn. They suddenly mean bad things to you.

People are telling you right and left that you are a bad person, which goes back to those early experiences with homophobia that formed the first fundamental layers of your being, of your personality. Your friends start to die, which causes a lot of grief. You have intense anxiety about your own future. You feel cut off from any long-term involvement with other people. Life seems pretty bleak because you think you're going to die, and to top it off, they start giving you poison to counteract the virus that's inside of you."

"Is that why you don't have your T cells monitored?"

"Definitely. That's why I stay away from it. That's why I don't get involved in all that stuff. And that's why Kyle and I decided we were not going to get tested. We weren't going to get into that."

Some of the media's shortcomings were understandable. News is a commodity, and death and disaster make much better copy than stories of survival. But the media weren't the only enemies. Despite mounting evidence to the contrary, health professionals everywhere spun a few statistical projections into proclamations that HIV was 100 percent fatal. These proclamations were issued at professional conference after conference for over a decade. Those who were entrusted with our care couldn't seem to refrain from pronouncing our deaths. Perhaps professionals on the conference circuit forgot that they saw only the sick ones. Perhaps they did not have adequate outlets for their own grief. Perhaps it was because they were academics and most of their "patients" came from journal articles. In my more sarcastic moods I thought they were bored with their lives, watched too many medical soap operas, or projected their need for drama onto their work. Most of the time I understood that the doomsday pronouncements helped maintain the power and resources that all professions accumulate during a perceived crisis on their protected turfs. This is not to imply conscious malfeasance on the part of those health professionals who managed to shed their scientific skepticism without shedding their scientific cloaks or persona. However, the public should never forget that professionals have a tendency to emphasize and perpetuate their own importance, authority, and advantage during crisis situations.

The power of the medical profession in the lives of everyday people is often experienced without being consciously understood. But Eric understood power dynamics. His analysis of the modern doctor's office reflected his deep distrust of physicians and is a good example of how many people might experience an office visit.

"Think about what happens when you go into a doctor's office. You are dealing with crucial issues, with life and death. Enter a person who has been given all the magical powers that our society bestows on anybody. They're almost religious. He is wearing—usually he, male authority—is wearing a white robe, you know. Wash your hands and stuff like that. The power dynamics are that you're coming in and asking for divination. You are being told what your status is, what your condition is. You're nervous because your very integrity as a person is threatened. Then you're told that you're near death, and it's given the full weight that our society can give it."

Once again, it was extremely difficult to get Eric to move away from his cultural critique to his personal story. I objected to his description of the doctor's office visit by saying that would not be true for me, in the hope that he would further describe what was true for him.

"Well, you're a nurse and an insider. More than that, nurses have a definite institutional and ideological stance against doctors, so you are much more defended. I'm a sociologist. I've thought about these issues, too. I'm also pretty defended, but imagine those people who aren't, who subscribe to the dominant ideology of doctors. They are extremely defenseless."

"I agree with you, Eric. I think that your description is very important and adequately captures the way a lot of people feel. But I'm wondering whether you, as Eric, could have substituted the word I for everything you said. Or are you detached from that picture you just drew? Are you vulnerable in the doctor's office, being there in front of the male authority, being scared about all this? Is that why you, as Eric, don't go, don't have your T cells monitored?"

"Yes, yes, yes. Yes, I don't do it because I do feel vulnerable. I saw how vulnerable I got when I did get tested. I was really scared for a while. I thought, oh my God, I'm going to die. It wasn't because I was afraid of the AIDS virus. It was because I had crossed the line and entered that whole reality. I was afraid I wasn't going to be strong enough to counter it.

"In 1985 I was actually part of a very small minority who did know they were positive. I don't know if you remember. Back then there was social pressure not to get tested. The *Sentinel*, the *New York Native* had these big huge headlines, 'Don't Take the Test.' Actually Kyle and I had talked about it. We thought it was dangerous to take the test because it would pull you more into that negative, labeling, mass-hysteria stuff of the dangerous medical world. We viewed the test and the whole medical model as hostile toward gay men. I saw the whole thing, the whole AIDS conception and the test and the labeling process, as an attack, an offensive, like in a war. I knew that a lot of gay men were succumbing to it. I knew that the testing, which had just been started, was one of the more potent weapons of this whole onslaught.

"As you know, I write about this stuff and I think about it. So I thought to be really effective, I would have to undergo it myself—to see how it was affecting gay men and what type of issues it brought up and what type of self-imaging it created and ideas it produced about one's self and one's relation to the world. So I sort of volunteered myself, so I could better analyze it and write about it. It sounds strange, but that was very conscious. I guess I also simply wondered if I was or wasn't because I was very healthy and hadn't had any symptoms that I knew of. But I didn't tell Kyle that I got tested because I thought he was more vulnerable to all that than I was and I didn't want to pull him into that with me."

▼▼▼

When Kyle finally did find out that Eric had been tested, he was furious, not because Eric took the test, but because he had pretended for so long that he had not. Duplicity or inconsistency became evident in several areas in my interactions with Eric. He expressed beliefs both in condoms and in knowledgeable "superpatients," but he was neither a superpatient nor a consistent condom user. Duplicity gave Eric the ability to live in more than one world, but it also required that he live in more than one world, and that did not always go smoothly for him.

"I don't have a doctor. You know, I don't do all that. I kind of figure it out. I talk to my friends who are knowledgeable about medicine, and then I make my own decisions. I use the student health center. They try to educate you and make you totally responsible for your own health care. They refuse to play the role of the shaman.

"What I personally feel is that the status and the role of doctors and the medical profession need to be reduced to those of a plumber. Medical information and education in the general public need to be increased so that everybody knows enough about commonsense medical and health issues to figure things out and make their own decisions, like Kyle and I do. Then go to a mere plumber-type of person, a doctor, to like prescribe the stuff or to set the bone or to do the T cells or whatever. Until the roles become that equal, I think getting involved with the medical world is dangerous."

"One of the nurse's jobs is to attenuate or bridge those unequal roles. We need a supernurse to accomplish it sometimes."

"Basically what we need is a superpatient, which, now that we're talking about it, might be what's happening in the gay community. I mean, God, do we know a lot about health. You know, Kyle and I have decided that we don't need doctors to a large extent. We just don't. We can figure it out. We even go to *DSM III*—no, that's the psychological one, we go to the—

"*PDR?*"

"—*PDR* and look it up ourselves."

Eric was not a superpatient. He had not made himself very knowledgeable about drugs or lab values and was not very familiar with the epidemiological research on HIV. Clinical AIDS nurses recognize these superpatients easily. Eric may be one someday, but wasn't one then. In his rush to equalize the power differential between doctors and patients, Eric forgot that some HIV-positive people were not any more interested in becoming superknowledgeable about HIV, and the diagnosis, monitoring, and treatment of its associated conditions, than he was. Although Eric believed in figuring it all out for himself, he was nonetheless plagued with anxiety over minor symptoms and frequently asked me for diagnoses, which I was never able to provide. This was another instance where his ideology didn't seem to be working for him.

At the same time, Eric's critique of medicine created a double bind. The physician must not be a shaman, but the medical establishment is blamed for having developed a singular, biological understanding of health and disease. On the one hand, Eric expected physicians to function as "plumbers." On the other, he tended to favor psychosocial approaches over biological ones, if only to even the score. In 1992 when Kyle and I were talking about whether he should take antivirals or medicine to prevent pneumocystis, Eric got furious because I was adjusting my recommendation based on an emerging understanding of what was important to Kyle, how Kyle viewed his situation. Eric's expectation was that health professionals would stick to "science"— even though we had had countless discussions about the dangers of scientism and the error in applying population findings to individuals without regard to the special characteristics of the individual. Eric's ideal for how AIDS might have been managed sounded strangely scientific at first.

▼▼▼

"If, in the beginning, AIDS was never invented, and it was simply a matter of a virus, and everyone kept their heads, and it didn't grow into the huge phenomenon that it did, then I would be more amenable to taking AZT or something else to deal with it. That scenario could have been wear a condom, treat everybody nicely, take AZT if it's warranted—not that big of a deal. I think the only real answer to AIDS is condoms. Condoms could have been introduced into the gay lifestyle a lot more calmly than they were in the early '80s. But instead it all became a big deal, a huge deal. It is one of the main battlegrounds in our society right now. It has the weight of the Reformation. It has the weight of religious war."

"Do you think that condoms could have been introduced without AIDS?"

"Yes. I do."

"How?"

"Just a general awareness that we live in a biological world, that sex has its risks, that if you love yourself and other people you minimize those risks. It's as simple as that. It didn't need this heavy-duty AIDS stuff. It didn't need an epidemic of worldwide proportions. It didn't need this medicalization of the entire gay community and gay lifestyle. All it needed was some care and some self-love. That's all it needed."

"When did condoms enter into your awareness?"

"Relatively soon at this point. After I came back to San Francisco."

"They were using condoms in New York in 1982?"

"No. Actually, Nick was the first guy who used them on me."

"So did you demand condoms from there on out?"

"No. Half the time."

"About half the time?"

"Okay. So then the next thing was that I came back to San Francisco and—"

In his own life not even AIDS had created sufficient impetus for him to use condoms consistently. In fact, Eric did none of this with anything approaching the fervor of a religious war, unless by religious war he meant a war of ideas. Even Eric's preferred, metaphorless answer to the AIDS crisis, "Wear a condom, treat people nicely, take AZT if warranted," was safely tucked away in the unreal condition of the future. For several years Eric was somehow excused from condom duties on the battleground of bodily experiences. The body may be "believed in," but like most people Eric tended to take it for granted unless it manifested problems.

I felt that Eric was simultaneously abandoning the body to biomedicine while rejecting biomedical interventions. For the next twenty minutes we argued about the function of medical technology. Today I have finally come to recognize that medical technology is never neutral. But during this conversation with Eric I argued that, even though laboratory values such as T-cell and hemoglobin levels had metaphoric meanings for people, they could nonetheless be understood as neutral technological pieces of information to interpret within the context of individual situations. He disagreed.

"Information does not come in a vacuum. Those laboratory values fall into a structured field of power relations. You get that information within the context of doctor-patient relationships, in the context of the whole medical, authoritative ideology. From what's been written about T cells, it seems to me that it's a manifestation of our technological fetishism with numbers. I think the same information can be experientially determined by how you feel, by how fit you are, by how well you can exercise. We mistrust that because it's not numbers and it's not technical. It's experiential; it's feeling. It's not left-brained. I think you can get the same information by looking at the texture of the skin, the color of the eyes, the state of your bowels, you know, all this type of stuff. You don't need to get hooked into that techno-, numerical, male-dominance-of-the-environment type of thing. You can do it in a whole other realm, which is what I prefer to do. Maybe you can double-check it every once in a while by doing the minimum lab tests possible, which I've actually done. Every once in a while I get my CBC [complete blood count] or whatever it's called done. They have been fine, up until now. Again, even if your T cells are low, I don't know what you are going to do. I don't think taking poison is a very good idea."

"So would you say that ACT-UP's diatribe against the Burroughs Wellcome Company is totally misguided?"[6]

"Totally."

"A good example of Foucault's resistance movements serving the very power structures they seek to undermine?"

"Completely. It reinforces techno-authority. It reinforces that we're all dying. It reinforces the whole medicalization of gays. It shifts the issue away from the more interesting and fundamental problem: male authority destroying the world. I think the stress overwhelmingly should be on having a balanced life."

"What is a balanced life?"

"Eating well, being happy, getting touched, having sex, feeling good about yourself, feeling good about others, you know, basic stuff. In our society that's very hard to do. So instead of putting so much energy into the techno-medical aspect of everything, put energy into making this a functional, livable society. If all those people who put so much life energy and so much expertise and intelligence and care into the medical aspect of things would put that into social activism, into creating a new society, into criticizing our society and trying to come up with solutions at the same time; if all those people who dealt with things in a medical way worked in a social-activist way instead, I think that everybody's general health would improve. Again, not just of gays but of everybody. A healthier society is impossible without a more workable society, and that means reducing alienation, anger, violence, drug addiction—all those things which cause ill health. We live in a society that basically doesn't function and needs to be revamped."

"See, I agree with all that. What I disagree with is that you can get all the information by looking at the color of your eyes and the texture of your skin. I also disagree that quantification is purely a manifestation of male, rational thinking. To me your position on the T cell seems like the same position someone would take against looking at anything under a microscope or through a telescope. It's simply, I mean, I'm going to argue with you that it is absolutely neutral. It is simply another lens."

"I don't see how you can argue that because, again, it's in the context of a structured field of power relations. One could envision a time and a place where it is just another lens, just more information, and just another technique, but it's not, right now. Not within the system we live in, within the society we live in."

▼ ▼ ▼

It still seemed to me that Eric was unnecessarily ceding useful scientific technology to the evil, male-dominated medical industry. However, the real difficulty may have been my own discomfort with my role as a nurse. If I had no power to alter the context in which antibody results and T-cell counts were received, if I had no power to help people interpret them despite the "structured systems of power," my role as a nurse would seem almost impossible. I decided to push one more time.

▼ ▼ ▼

"I'm sorry, Eric, but I think your analysis winds up handing the body and the physical and the biological over to the medical establishment. I guess that I want to reassert that it never belonged to them in the first place."

"That's a good point. That's a very good point."

"Society created the technology that lets us count T cells. Peasant farmers fed the cities where this technology was born. It's a product of human culture. It's not inherently bad, and it doesn't really belong to the corporate class."

"I agree with you. I think that is a very interesting and valid point. I do think I'm in danger of ceding the body, or giving the body over and forgetting about it. I'm not in principle opposed to the use of pharmaceuticals. It's just hard to find any that are safe—safe in the sense of being outside power relations, outside the framework of intervention with poisons. It's hard to find pharmaceuticals based on an attitude of bringing things into balance."

"Well, the virus isn't safe."

"Well, I'm sorry, but viral stuff seems to be a very murky area. I don't know why I don't have that concern with bacteria, but retroviruses, viruses, seem to be—I don't know very much about them, but they just seem to me to be open to a lot of interpretations."

Today we tend to think of scientific knowledge as exploding, but advances in health care tend to occur along a few technological and economically profitable paths. In the health sciences knowledge is not exploding in all directions. Many of the basic questions about viruses are still unanswered. Viruses still hang out in a vague realm between life and inanimate objects. Even though this "murky" virus seems to have killed a lot of people, many are surviving with the virus much longer than was expected, and some without pharmaceutical intervention. For Eric, the biotechnological aspect of health care had been overemphasized to the point where he would need to "actively fight against it" in order to achieve a balance.

I thought Eric was right about that in 1990, and I am even more convinced today. We have put almost all of our efforts into fighting a virus and almost nothing into learning how to strengthen the immune system. The *Time* 1996 Man of the Year thinks this is the proper state of affairs. "It's the virus, stupid," is the word from Dr. David Ho. Personally, I hope Dr. Ho is right and both Eric and I are wrong. I'd be more than happy to take an effective pharmaceutical cocktail—a silver bullet—and not have to depend on going to the gym, taking vitamins, reducing stress, getting enough sleep, eating regularly, going to the acupuncturist, or avoiding alcohol. I wondered if Eric would even be willing to take a silver bullet should one ever be developed.

▼ ▼ ▼

"If they do find the silver bullet, HIV will be suddenly demystified. It will no longer carry any of its social weight. It will no longer be a terrain. I would probably take the silver bullet and go on to the next thing. Once a silver bullet is produced, this battle is over. It's a moot point and you go on. But it's not at that point yet. It's really like a paradox."

"That's the problem with silver bullets. They increase our reliance on biological-technological understandings about health."

"It's like we got away this time."

"Again."

"Again, but it doesn't mean that they were right. Not taking a silver bullet would be a silly reason to die, a silly way to die. But it's not at that point yet, and it's ridiculous to act as if it is. It's just not productive. Even if you do take the silver bullet, the danger is that you forget about the social issues. The social issues will remain the same and a new epidemic will arise.[7] Western civilization, and the world, for that matter, has relied on these silver bullets for too long. We are running out of silver. We can't get by on that anymore. We can't keep ignoring the social issues."

▼▼▼

In 1992 Eric did finally have his T cells drawn at the student health center. I went with him to the follow-up appointment because he was very anxious and frightened. On the way he said that he was going to tell the physician that he didn't want to know the results, but the physician announced that Eric's T-cell count was 400 before even saying hello. Eric was grateful that I had gone with him because the interaction was stressful, and it took him some time to process what having 400 T cells meant to him. Within a week, however, he developed a kind of Marxist indignation (or simply a competitive stance) toward anyone who had a higher T-cell count than he did. Four years later when his first viral load count came back at less than 10,000 (the best result possible at the time), a few of us couldn't resist a bit of contemptuous jealousy at his greater power and worth.

Over time the medical technology lost some of the metaphoric power it had once held for Eric. Today he incorporates laboratory and epidemiological data into his own emerging understanding of HIV. As an academic and social critic, resisting the dominant medical and social understandings of HIV/AIDS came naturally for Eric. As a person with HIV, developing an understanding of what HIV and its associated medical technology meant in his own life took more time.

In 1998 Eric is still healthy. His T-cell count has remained stable in the 250–400 range, and his viral load fluctuates between 10,000 and

36,000. Even though he monitors both T cells and viral loads, he continues to refuse the antiviral cocktail. As a result, Eric has endured the condescending glances and remarks from his physicians. Convinced of their own superior intelligence and authority, they could not comprehend why Eric agreed to monitoring while refusing treatment.

In 1998 when Eric told his new physician that he had never done and was not interested in antivirals, the physician assumed a more open-minded attitude.

"Well," said the physician, looking up from his chart. "As it turns out, you were right. The question now is whether you're still right."

The Heresy of Holism: Jason

Jason and his lover, Kim, moved to San Francisco in 1988, shortly after my lover, Duckus, had died. Both designers, they rented a modest apartment, shared a car, and dreamed of building a house in the Bahamas. Suspicious of consumerism and its associated values, they shared a kind of airy-fairy cosmic consciousness that cared about people and the environment. Jason was forever on guard against mucus-producing dairy, cancer-inducing additives, and any chemical that did not make people high. Jason and Kim soon attracted a large circle of friends and became a kind of first family to San Francisco's muscle queens. At our Christmas festivities Jason sang melody and Kim sang tenor.

This couple knew how to treat a grieving widower and often had me over for beautiful but simple organic dinners. Chopsticks were the rule, but they kindly obliged my preference for a knife and fork. A few times I tried to wash the dinner dishes and endured a bitchy barrage about how much water I used, how much water I splashed, and why I didn't fill the second sink for rinsing. Later I discovered that none of their friends helped with the dishes, and I learned to watch Kim light the candles in the living room, where Jason would eventually join us.

Jason was a very attractive man in his early thirties. Except for noticeably enlarged lymph nodes in the back of his neck that had popped up a few years before, he presented a picture of radiant health. One night after dinner Jason and Kim mentioned that neither of them had been tested for HIV. Further probing revealed that they weren't practicing safe sex either, reasoning that neither of them wanted to live if the other one died. I literally screamed at their "foolishness" and strongly encouraged both of them to take the test. As it turned out, I was not the only one pushing them in this direction. When they finally succumbed to the community pressure in 1989, Jason's test was positive and Kim's was negative.

A year later I wondered whether we had made a mistake in encouraging this couple to get tested. Initially, of course, we felt that we had saved Kim's life. They started practicing safe sex after taking the test. Yet despite all Jason's positive thinking and airy-fairy holism, he seemed more frightened than the rest of us were. And despite Jason's distrust of Western medicine, he seemed to be more obsessed with his T-cell counts than anyone I knew.

We made an appointment to talk about Jason's approach to HIV on February 1, 1990. When I arrived at their house, Jason was almost out of his body with excitement over recently acquired tickets to the Saint party in New York City. The Saint had been America's preeminent gay disco. It was already closed but occasionally resurrected itself with a megaparty that attracted the international gay party set—middle-class queens, mostly, but few with more than thirty-three-inch waistlines.

As we sat at the breakfast table overlooking the San Francisco skyline, I let him gloat for a while before we started talking about his first year as an "HIV positive" in San Francisco. In many previous discussions, Jason had made it clear that he was extremely suspicious of the medical establishment and of AZT, so his opening statement really surprised me.

▼▼▼

"I decided to go on AZT."

"What! You're going to do AZT? When did you decide that?"

"Yesterday. We were having dinner with Sam and Rhoda, and I decided in the restaurant, in the bathroom. Something happened in there. First of all, Lance is doing it, and he's fine. Then I found out that Sam's doing it, too. I didn't even know. He doesn't talk about it very much, but his T cells went down. Plus there was that article about insurance companies and the FDA's approving AZT on the front page of the *Examiner*. Obviously, the general consensus is that AZT is useful.

"It's not that I have faith in the FDA, but I've been asking people who've started AZT what their T cells were. Most of them say 300 or 400, and they are all freaked out. Jesus, maybe I should be more concerned, but I'm not. And see, that's my struggle. I feel fine. I feel healthy.

I think if I was in danger or something, I would know. I'm just that type of person. But I decided to start AZT if my T cells go down again. I'm not going to struggle anymore."

▼▼▼

The year had not been easy for Jason, but the struggles had actually begun before he and Kim had moved to San Francisco.

"I went to the doctor at the Gay Men's Health Crisis [GMHC] in New York. They suggested that I get tested, but I said I wasn't interested. They told us that we should be having safe sex with each other, and we said that we'd never had safe sex and weren't about to start doing that. The counselor mentioned that since we were having three-ways, we should definitely be having safe sex. That's what started me thinking that maybe I was living in a bit of dreamworld.

"And then the Saint closed. That really shook me up. I've never really talked about it, but the Saint closing was the single most blatant statement that our community was dying. So many people who used to go there were dead or dying or sick. Most of the guys we knew from the Saint had lost two lovers—Robert, Jack, Anthony. One night Jack told me he had seventeen friends who were sick.

"Then we moved to San Francisco, and everything seemed to be quite fine until I got sick in November. Remember how I was coughing up all this stuff and didn't get over it? I wasn't going to the doctor. I was just trying to deal with it. So that's basically how I came to take the test in February of 1989. It's amazing that I waited so long to get tested, but for me it was a major breakthrough. None of my friends in Boston has ever been tested. Even George still hasn't been tested. I find that odd when I think about it, but it's different back there than it is here. I think it's denial. Grand-scale denial. We're much more AIDS conscious in San Francisco. This community is incredible. We're totally aware. I mean, what do you do when you open the paper at night? I look for AIDS first in every headline. I flip through the paper and look for any news about AIDS, anything that says, 'AIDS,' or 'gay,' or 'HIV-related,' or anything. They don't live like that."

▼▼▼

That wasn't how people in my house lived either. I had already lost two lovers, but unlike Jason, I never connected the closing of several bars, bathhouses, and discos to the death of the whole community. Every year the Gay Pride Parade seemed just as crowded as it had ever been. There were still as many pictures of hunks up on the "wall of shame" at Castro and Market Streets. It never once occurred to me that the whole gay community might be dying. Heterosexuals were producing gays at the same rate that they always had, and even if it killed half of us, 99 percent of the lesbians and 50 percent of the gay men would still constitute a community. But Jason wasn't talking about a theoretical gay community. He was taking about a specific community of men he knew and loved.

Moving from Boston to San Francisco was more difficult for him than I had understood. Jason had actually avoided San Francisco in the mid-1980s because the city was "so depressed." By 1990 we had "learned how to party again," but much had changed. The newspapers were full of AIDS stories, and even though Jason didn't believe much of what he read, he was still anxious for the news. His friends had changed, too. In addition to talking about parties and men, they were now discussing their T cells or planning the next memorial service. His friends in Boston were still suspicious of the HIV test, whereas most of his San Francisco friends had taken it. However, Jason had not altogether rejected the Boston approach. According to Jason, his Boston friends had avoided testing because they didn't want to "buy into the consciousness of the disease," and that was something he had to fight against in San Francisco. I asked what buying into the consciousness of the disease was all about.

"Battling against the thought that you'll eventually die from AIDS is like swimming upstream. The hundredth monkey has not yet thought that HIV is a manageable condition. We're still living in the belief that we're all going to die from it. It's a mental concept. I wonder how long people would live if they weren't tested at all. They might live twenty or thirty years and just go through normal illnesses and get better because they believe that they'll get better. Now I watch my T cells go down, and I think, uh-oh, they might never go back up again. With that attitude, our chances are cut in half. I really believe that getting tested is not for everybody because you have to be willing and able to overcome your fears."

▼▼▼

I wondered how Jason's battle was going and whether there was any-thing that might be done to help him. I wondered if his only weapon against fear was the belief that not everyone with HIV would die from AIDS. A number of his friends shared that belief—perhaps not as fer-vently as Jason did, but with less apparent anxiety. Even so, people were dropping dead and it wasn't all because of their minds. When I asked Jason how we might create a consciousness of hope without denying the fact that we were living with a deadly virus, Jason jumped into a discus-sion of support groups that revealed a serious belief in mental powers.

▼ ▼ ▼

"I don't think that any of those support groups really work. It's like a bunch of people getting together who feel that they've got to somehow struggle to survive. I don't even want to think that I have to survive. Once you get down to the level of finding out you've got something, once you start fighting to survive, then you've put into existence that there's something that's trying to kill you."

I thought Jason was taking the positive-thinking mind-over-matter philosophy too far. I told him I figured that chances were greater than 50/50 that I would die from AIDS, and I wasn't putting anything "into existence" by saying so. He exploded and we argued for a while.

"Well, that's just what I've been trying to not figure. I can't under-stand why you'd want to think that! Because deep down you know that whatever you believe is what you're creating in your life. So don't believe that. A million people are HIV positive, and so far only a tenth of those are sick. If we all believe we'll eventually die from AIDS, then we certainly will."

"I don't believe I'll die from AIDS. I'm just saying my chances are rather high. What else am I going to die from? I'm thirty-seven years old."

"You could die of old age, for heaven's sake. You could never die of AIDS. You could never even contract it. As soon as we find out we're HIV positive, we just wait until the day that something starts happen-ing to us. More than any other disease, I think you have to have a posi-tive attitude with HIV. You can't sit around thinking that you're going to get sick."

"My argument with you is that you say that you're not afraid of dying and I think that you are. You can't stare it in the face and say, 'This could kill me.'"

"No, I'm not afraid of it. I just don't want to die right now. I'm not done. I haven't done all I want to do. I think the ones who focus on sickness and dying the least are the healthiest ones to face death. Remember how we always used to say that perhaps the thing to do was to get into harmony with the virus? Maybe we should think, 'Okay, you're living here, and as soon as I die, you're dead, so we just have to live here together.' I try to do that—try to be at peace with it. I thought I would be a major stressed-out mess. I don't know, maybe I have been. My friends would know better. But I don't think so. I basically deal with it better than I thought I ever would and better than most people I know. A lot of people get tested and it's a tragedy. But take Bart. To me, he's the ultimate example of how to deal with HIV. He's known he's been positive for four years, and it doesn't even affect him the least bit."

"Why should it? He's got 900 T cells and is totally healthy," I replied.

"So am I! I'm healthy, too! My doctor says 'T cells, T schmells. You're not a T cell.' What about healthy people who don't have HIV? How do you know that their T cells don't go down to 100 when they get something and then go back up to 1,000? They don't monitor T cells in all those people, so that could be a common occurrence. This is the problem with an unknown situation like this, but we start living in fear and thinking it's something bad.

"Like right now, I'm sitting here thinking I have to make some effort in the next two weeks to get my T cells up. I have to start getting my rest. I have to not be stressed. Let me see, maybe I shouldn't go to work today and rest instead. But if I don't, then I'll go in tomorrow and things will be really tense. Then I think maybe I'll quit my job, but maybe I can't because it might affect my T cells, and that would mean I'd have to get on AZT, and I don't know how I'll react to AZT. So everything is based around my fucking T cells, including building the house in Hawaii! Which is ridiculous! My doctor says not to worry about my T cells, but I'm getting a lot of outside pressure here. I get barraged with information—from my doctors, from you, and from all of my other friends who love me."

▼ ▼ ▼

Jason had tried to avoid the numbers game altogether, but once he succumbed to blood testing, retreat was impossible. T cells came to have a number of meanings for him, not all of which were consistent with each other. On the one hand, T cells were meaningless and artificial definitions of health. Jason's 300 T cells didn't make him any less healthy than Bart, who had 900. His lymphadenopathy, night sweats, and chronic upper respiratory infections didn't make him any less healthy than Bart either, and Bart had no symptoms at all.

On the other hand, Jason thought that T cells were a "good measure of viral progression," and he also felt challenged to raise them. He wasn't the only one who felt this pressure. Though nobody expected people to raise their own T cells, many felt responsible for doing just that. The sense of personal responsibility for raising one's T cells was not just confined to people with "holistic" attitudes like Jason's. In 1995 an old friend came up to me at the gym and asked if I thought his workout would affect his T-cell count. At first I thought he was asking whether workouts were good for people with HIV, and I was all set to encourage him to keep it up. But then it became clear he was having blood drawn later in the day. He wanted today's workout to raise today's T-cell count. It wasn't at all uncommon for men in my community to attempt to raise their T cells a few days prior to having them drawn.

Others—and fewer in number I would guess—wanted to know the worst news as soon as possible in order to make treatment decisions at the most efficacious time. This is the rational model. The medical purpose for monitoring T cells is either to facilitate treatment decisions or to document an individual history that might facilitate treatment decisions in the future. However, people don't always interpret their blood tests within the medical model. T cells also indicate prognostic probabilities and therefore function as a measure of one's health and even of one's life.

One of the only ways to get out from under the enormous pressure and sense of responsibility for low T-cell counts was to periodically assert that they were meaningless. For men like Jason, T-cell counts tended to function as report cards or tests for which one had to cram. The ambivalence these men felt about T cells was similar to that of students who cram or hope for good grades while at the same time maintaining that grades are meaningless. Jason had asserted that testing was not for everyone. I wondered whether the test and T-cell monitoring were good ideas for him and asked why he was having his T cells tested and what he was going to do with the information.

"I'm doing them because, in addition to other values, I think they are a proven barometer of the immune system's strength and the progression of the virus. It gives me information that I believe is actually valuable. I'm going to program it into the way that I feel and then see how I'll use it to deal with treating the situation. My T cells have dropped about 150 points in the last year. Now they've gone down even more. They're in the 300 range. My percentage has also gone down. So there's a general tendency for my counts to go down. I have to figure that all the research that's being done is not total bullshit. I don't want to let it go to the point where I'm beyond help, you know.

"AZT is what I have my doubts about. I feel very strongly that I should not be doing AZT. It's very toxic. My body is not going to deal with it very well. I have a hard enough time with pentamidine. My whole face and shoulders all break out. This is with a half a dose of pentamidine. It's very toxic, too."

Jason gave the logical response for why he was monitoring his T cells, but he still felt conflicted by the whole process. There were at least two good reasons that he felt this conflict, neither of which I fully appreciated at the time. First, the only medical option for a low T-cell count in 1990 was AZT, and Jason had grave doubts about that particular drug. Second, there was an enormous pressure in the community for people like Jason to accept AZT because that was the only offensive weapon we had.

People made different decisions about when to start taking AZT. For some it was when the count dropped below 500; others thought it was best to wait until their T cells hit 200. In 1990 my own magic number was 300. But Jason didn't argue that people should wait until the number dropped to any particular level. That would have involved negative thinking. Instead, Jason argued that the only offensive weapon we had was worthless (or worse, that it would backfire). Jason's argument infringed on our positive thinking, and he was outnumbered. From Jason's point of view, his friends and I were pushing not only poison, but also poison produced by an establishment he mistrusted.

"You view it differently than I do because you live in that medical world and I don't. I've never had a trust of all of that. Plus I mistrust who backs it. You know, the fact that you push it is different, but it's being backed by a whole group of organizations that I mistrust completely.

"If the FDA is recommending that more people do AZT, maybe it's because they want more of us to be dead. They know people are hyper about finding something to do. There's such a hype about AZT because it's the only thing so far. So they'll spend years slowly going through the process of getting everyone to take AZT, but in the end everyone is going to die from the AZT. They're all going to slowly break down their immune systems and kill off their bone marrow cells. Eventually, they'll realize they can't keep doing AZT for time immemorial. With the high dose you could last, what, fourteen months to two years? Now with a lower dose maybe you can last three years, maybe even five years. But it's just a dead end. I just would rather not get involved in anything that is backed by the government or the FDA in any way. I believe that they are ultimately responsible for the whole epidemic in the first place. They are the cause of it. They created it. They have let it run rampant. And they are still to this day.

"Now Reagan's just made his little commercial. And it was about children with AIDS. Who gives a fuck? I don't give a fuck about children with AIDS, actually," he said, laughing. "They're nothing compared to our community. We are devastated. So a few little children get AIDS, and they can all run around like the kid that fell in the well. Who gives a shit about that one little two year old that fell in the well? Millions of people are dying, and they make this whole big thing about the precious life of a child. But they can turn their back on the rest of us. That's the real truth. That's where their hearts are really at. That's why I don't want to have anything to do with AZT and the government and the way that they back it."

One night Jason gave a similar speech as we were driving to the disco. Howard, a dreamboat of a guy who'd been suffering from AIDS for more than two years, interrupted him: "Burn your bra, girlfriend. You'll feel better after."

▼▼▼

It was difficult for people with HIV not to feel anger and alienation in 1990. Most in the federal government couldn't even bring themselves to say the word *AIDS*. When that became unavoidable, both health care professionals and gay leaders worked to sanitize the disease for the general public by downplaying its distinctly gay male demographics. I always saw myself apart from the medical mainstream, both as a clinician and as an academic. However, friends such as Eric and Jason saw me as representing establishment views that they found oppressive.

As I reread Jason saying, "The fact that you push it—," I realize they were right. Since 1992 I've been arguing with those who are convinced that the only way to prevent AIDS is to fight HIV, but in 1990 I rarely challenged mainstream views like those of Matthew, Ron, or Brian. I argued with the heretics such as Eric and Jason, not because I thought their ideas were outrageous, but because I wanted to sort out the compelling logical arguments from the illogical ones. I had a vested interest in getting it right.

It was interesting to me that Jason talked freely about any problem with his physical or mental health, but unless the problem was "worrying too much," he almost never connected it to HIV. Most of the time he linked health problems of any sort to other aspects of his life—too much stress, too much partying, or too many dairy products because he had to go to a birthday party. Most of Jason's decisions about health-related issues were made within a social context. Getting tested, monitoring T cells, taking AZT—even safe sex was couched in terms of what the rest of his friends were doing. Boston was in denial; San Francisco was very aware. Living in San Francisco forced Jason to face his HIV status, but he never mentioned that the move from Boston to San Francisco was also changing him.

Despite all the rhetoric about personal autonomy and individual choice in the academic community, when it comes to health care, validation from one's community is often essential. Professional therapeutic relationships are not a substitute for family, friendship, and community relationships. Jason was dealing with several simultaneous pressures. He felt pressured to raise his T cells and conflicted about what they meant. He wanted to be "aware" like his new group of friends in San Francisco, even as these new friends were challenging some of his holistic attitudes. In addition, Jason was experiencing conflict between his sexual fantasies and his idea of what sex should be like.

▼▼▼

"In Boston we hadn't even heard of safe sex until 1984. Things have changed so much. At first my group stayed mostly unaffected and we still did our thing. We hardly knew anybody who was sick. We did know a couple in Boston who used to throw a lot of parties. They had a third lover, Hal, who died of pneumonia in 1986, and I was getting that old attitude—that only the promiscuous ones were dying. But that was definitely the case with these three. Hal had a different partner every two days. He was really very active. They were always throwing big parties and orgies at their house. They were the wild people.

"Of course, I had sex with all of them, but it didn't faze me. I didn't think it would ever mean anything. It's weird how I did that. I don't know if that was denial or not, but back then there was a general theory that buying into AIDS had to do with issues in your head, and a lot of it was guilt. Very early theories around the whole Louise Hay thing were coming out, and we really believed all that. Of course, we were all doing Ecstasy every weekend, so it was normal for us to believe in being loving. And all the people we knew who had been sick were really in a state of being down on themselves, full of sexual guilt and nonacceptance. Take Thomas, for instance. He was the most negative person I had ever known. He didn't get along with anybody, fought with everybody. He was completely guilt-ridden and guilt-tripped by his parents. His crowd was always hanging out at the Mine Shaft [a New York City gay bar with a notorious back room]. They liked to be abused or mentally dominated and even got a little bit more negated. All of that was coming out in the way they lived their lives. Some of the things that people do are just not life affirming, are not exalting.

"I think our sex life tends to be that way. You know, Kim's and my sex life is very much based on fantasy. It's not one-on-one loving each other. I'm such a control person. My whole life exists in the realm of me being in charge of things. That's what my field of work is. I'm the great organizer. I'm the one who figures out how to do things and build buildings and break down all the pieces and put all the pieces in order and see that it all comes together. It's my whole life. So I like to be in a position where I'm not in control sexually, and all of our fantasies revolve around dominating-type things, which tend to be master-slave things and stuff on that level. To me, that's not healthy because it's not about loving the other person. Sex has this total way of releasing. But as far as the domination or S&M or leathery-type sex goes, I just don't think it's healthy. I never have thought it was very healthy. I don't understand why there should be any sort of mental degradation or physical pain connected with loving. It does not make sense to me at all.

"I think a lot of it comes from guilt—feeling guilty that you're gay. Wanting to be dominated by a couple of big daddy types who poke your lights out is a sheer example of the feeling that you're not responsible for what you're doing. It's denial. It leaves me very empty. It's not fulfilling. I'm at a point of wanting to change that in my life, and I make a major effort. What's happened is that we don't have even half as much sex as we used to. We'll go for a month or maybe have sex once every two weeks, but when we do, we actually connect with each other, and I feel a lot better. But see, we're into this addictive pattern of what we get turned on by—more raunchy, seedy sex.

"I really don't feel like it's okay, but I must think it's okay since I do it all the time. And therein lies the big problem—I'm continually doing things I don't think are okay. I either have to make it okay, or I have to stop doing it. But the bottom line is that I feel I need more love. I need more real love, more trust, more real faith. We have a lot of issues that keep coming up for us."

▼ ▼ ▼

Like most of us, Jason did things he didn't think were "okay," things that weren't consistent with his ideas about life. Sex and AIDS had a moral equivalent for Jason. To some extent, Jason thought people brought AIDS on themselves or created it out of a lack of self-love. Perhaps bad things such as AIDS create a certain quantity of blame that has to go somewhere. Though it is certainly best to keep blame and shame off one's own dress, this is hard for the girl who wants to dance by open fires and then sleep under the stars. Jason had somehow managed to play with the bad boys without being a bad boy. He could get high on Ecstasy and dance all night with loving friends, perhaps with a three-way afterward, but that was defined as having a good time. Taking crystal and having sex all night at the Mine Shaft were examples of being down on yourself, and Jason didn't do that. This is how Jason differentiated the "good boys" from "bad boys."

The tendency to differentiate oneself from those who are dying is widespread (Freud, Brown, Becker, Watney).[8] In the early days of AIDS many gay men looked around and concluded that it was only the hard-core party crowd that was getting sick. Often, these guys were the first to get sick. And even though Jason "had sex with them all," he was different because they were doing it every night and "all over town." When it became clear that both good boys and bad boys were coming down with AIDS, a new differentiation was required.

For Jason and many others like him, the central distinction between those who would live and those who would die was "self-love" and positive thinking. But Jason's "self-negating" sexual fantasies put him on the wrong side of his own differentiation. Jason could distinguish himself from the hard-core crowd on the basis of degree. But Jason's rule about self-love was much more exacting than his prohibition against excessive promiscuity. Jason's idea of himself as a New Age, full-of-love, sexy gay man was confronted by his erotic responses to masochistic fantasies. His body was natural. His ideology was holistic. His spirituality was loving. But he understood his sexual fantasies as the end product of wrong thinking, of internalized homophobia. The mind-body consciousness that had once provided some psychic protection against AIDS now threatened him with it. Jason's inability to keep "negative" thoughts out of his sex life was a constant reminder that his ability to control his own mind was limited. Jason had also started using his new San Francisco "awareness" of AIDS to differentiate himself from his friends in Boston.

"I'm obviously not totally into the mentality of my friends in Boston. They feel fine, so they're not doing anything. They're not being tested. So they're the ones who will suddenly find out that they have 65 T cells and come down with something. Whereas I'm at least monitoring. I'm just not choosing to take any aggressive antiviral action right now. I'm just choosing to try to have harmony. I have a lot of inner-peace things that I need to get together. When I start taking AZT, I'm going to have to deal with a new drug in my body as well.

"I'm actually doing lots of things. I went on St. John's wort, which has been very good. I was doing red clover for a while because it's real good to detoxify. When my T cells went down to 206, I told the acupuncturist 'I'm having my T cells done in a month, so we have to try to raise them.' He can usually tell if I've been eating right or drinking or getting stressed out based on my pulses."

Inner peace can be as hard to deal with as new treatments or medications such as AZT. However, holistic practices such as meditation and acupuncture are meant to affirm, balance, and support life, not raise T cells. When holistic practices are transformed into instrumental attempts to control the body, they often lose their positive effects. Perhaps that is why so much of the psychosocial research in HIV and cancer has not produced the unequivocal links between biopsychosocial phenomena that academics in the social sciences have come to expect. When Transcendental Meditation is done with the intention of prolonging life, it ceases to be transcendental and becomes yet another instance of instrumentalism. Visualizing white cells eating viruses may be motivated by fear one day and self-love the next; it may result in a sense of increased mastery and control or engender a sense of futility associated with a last-ditch effort. Mainstream researchers find it hard to understand or measure the intentions behind such health practices (if they bother to consider them at all). But when holistic approaches are used as means to control the body, they cease to be "holistic." In addition, such approaches encourage people like Jason to imagine themselves as being more powerful, more responsible, and more guilty than they really are.

"I think I'm basically very healthy. I eat right. I don't really drink all that much, and I'm not doing drugs anymore. But after my T cells went up to 368, I wasn't so careful. I started drinking again. We started going out on weekends and having a few margaritas here or there. And then I started smoking pot a little bit, and then there you go. My T cells dropped down to 240 again."

▼ ▼ ▼

Holistic health enthusiasts are not the only ones who try to differentiate their behavior from the "other" who is sick or dying. Rational people who are not themselves facing a life-threatening condition will often wonder how on earth people can continue smoking or drinking after being diagnosed with something like emphysema or heart disease. I've heard this reaction over and over from nurses and nursing students. People often forget that it's almost impossible to maintain a sense of crisis in a chronic situation, not that doing so would be healthy anyway. A medical diagnosis often seems a crisis to the one who hasn't been living with the diagnosis for years and years. Like so many people facing a life-threatening condition, especially one that moves as slowly as HIV often does, Jason was confronted with the nearly impossible task of maintaining his sense of who he was and what he believed while at the same time coping with huge changes in his life.

▼ ▼ ▼

"I don't think I could ever get the virus to die out of my system, but I really believe that if I get in harmony with the virus in my body, I could just live and live and live on. I just need to get healthier, to make my life more together, to create less and less stress, to work out more problems and things that bother me. For the first six months I used to think I would only live for two to three years. Remember? I was very tragic about it. Then somewhere along the line I started to realize that I was projecting that world, and that world was going to become my reality. I couldn't see beyond that. I used to see Tara [his niece] and I would think, I'm never going to see her grow up. She won't ever even remember me because I'll probably die when she's four or five. I don't remember people from when I was four or five. I thought about that a lot and finally asked myself why I wasn't thinking that I'd live for five more years. Just start to believe that for a while! Now I really believe that I will. Before it was just faith. I had to make myself think it. But now I really believe. Now I completely know it inside that I'm not going— I would be very surprised if I die of AIDS within the next two to three years."

"I would be very much surprised if you died of AIDS in three years. I would be very surprised."

"Why! I only have 240 T cells."

"Well, it takes longer than that."

"I would be surprised, too. I really believe I'll live for five more years. And so now I've started to project that I'll live for ten more years—or I'll live to be forty, which will be like, seven more years. And the more that you affirm that, you think, forty doesn't seem like very long; I should certainly be able to survive that long. In that process you realize how much you buy into dying without even thinking about it. I'm not even sick! Let's see. I was exposed in 1981. I was twenty-five. I would have survived for fifteen years, right?"

"I don't think there's any reason you shouldn't live to be forty."

▼ ▼ ▼

The optimism I expressed to Jason in 1990 reflected my desire to be more supportive. It also reflected my own hopes, expectations, and experience. These would soon change. Gabe's T cells plunged quickly and he died in 1991. Jason was fighting full-blown AIDS by 1993. By then I had seen significant variability in the patterns of life expectancy, including both long-term survival with low T cells and rapid declines leading to illness and death.

There were areas in Jason's life that contained not a shred of ambivalence or conflict, areas where he did indeed translate his thinking into the material world. He dreamed about living on an island and building a house together with Kim. Before the year was up, they broke ground. From San Francisco life led them briefly down a narrow windy road and a treacherous stretch of dirt that twisted through flowers and banana farms. There, perched on a cliff overlooking the sea, Jason manifested his dream, and died.

| 7 |

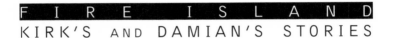

KIRK'S AND DAMIAN'S STORIES

Death itself carved out the decade of my thirties, taking three of my closest loved ones, but I never let a mortician set foot inside the house. God might decide when to take their lives, but I would decide when their bodies, their precious bodies that I had loved, soothed, and bathed, were ready to leave home for the last time.

Steve died in the morning and seemed to both brighten and frown after we put him into his best suit, so we blared Donna Summer, Gladys Knight, and Santa Esmeralda to assure him that he wasn't going to work. Duckus died in the early afternoon and had exhorted us to celebrate, not mourn, his death, so we bought balloons, played Music from the Heart over and over again, and ate a big dinner together in the same room with him. Gabe died deep in the night, so we gathered around his great bed, lit yet more candles, and blended our prayers with Fauré's sweet Requiem.

Once a nurse called the funeral home without telling us, and the morticians came unexpectedly. "We're not finished," I insisted, and sent them away. Death might come uninvited, but Charon himself would await our call and then remain outside at the curb. We, not strangers, would lift our friends and lovers from their beds and bear them out of their rooms, through the hallways and doorways, and down the stairs. Better for us to almost drop them than to watch strangers carry them off effortlessly. To undergird our efforts, we'd blare a cacophony of horns and drums on the stereo that would drive our little procession out onto the street, where the deads' ferry waited.

Some surge of ancient blood would press my own hands toward torching their pyres and crushing their bones. But we usually had less than ten days to write, direct, and produce a fitting memorial service, so we'd forgo the torching and the crushing, though it seemed to me the proper duty of a man.

Months or years later we would gather again and hold their ashes tightly in our hands before tossing them up like fireworks, the brighter grains gently falling as the lighter dust twisted up into the air like long-stemmed roses. Another handful would slip slowly through our fingers into that sacred space between the ocean and her sands. This was our obedience to the earth and the life that she gave. Thank you for the gift of this man. Thank you, thank you.

I never stopped loving Fire Island, and I returned again and again to remember love and death. My gaze meandered out across the Atlantic. Thirteen years ago this ocean had framed my first glimpse of eternity, pooled in Steve's brown eyes. Four years ago we had scattered his ashes here and this same ocean had swallowed everything up again. And still it lapped at this long white stretch of now-deserted beach.

This summer day in 1990 was almost over. The sun had crossed over to the bay side, and the boys were already at "tea," the late afternoon dance at the harbor. I dug my feet down to where the sand was cold and let my fingers crawl just beneath the warm surface. Nobody danced at tea anymore—just cruising and cocktails.

Might some of these tiny pebbles be Steve, tossed and polished by the ravenous surf? I liked the idea and stretched out to embrace as much beach as possible. Given the amount of fairy dust that had been scattered on this beach over the past several years, I was probably lying on the bones of a half dozen brothers.

I wondered whether Duckus's ashes should join the others. Fire Island hadn't enchanted him the way it had me, but the reason for his first and only trip was different from mine. Steve had directed that his ashes be spread on Fire Island, and he was still very much with us on our 1986 trip. Duckus and I hadn't taken a major vacation since getting together the summer before. I tried to fashion it into a honeymoon, but my attempt to celebrate love and death in the same place was not entirely successful.

Duckus, who grew up in Sparks, Nevada, had never been to New York. He'd been to Los Angeles only once. Ten years earlier at the age of twenty he had had a few rushed tours of second-string cities with the

Oakland Ballet, but those experiences had not molded him much. Duckus remained as sweet and suburban as Steve Richter had been sophisticated and cosmopolitan. We peered down at the city from the Empire State Building and strolled through Greenwich Village and Central Park, but it was the Circle Line cruise around Manhattan that coaxed out his biggest smiles.

When Steve's best friend, Sherman, a mensch if there ever was one, heard that Duckus would accompany me to "the island," he put two tickets for the Sea Plane on his Visa card. Sherman's generosity rumbled down the East River like an old VW van, winged over bridges, arched back across midtown, flew across Long Island, and floated us over to the yacht harbor at Fire Island Pines—a splendid way to move from Gotham to Paradise. A friend of Sherman's met us at the dock and lent us a wagon to help transport our bags. We had an upscale oceanside house to ourselves, courtesy of friends too sick to join us for the scattering. Duckus decided he would fly home before Steve's friends arrived. He was emphatic about my doing that part without him. I wanted so much for the heaven I had known on earth to show itself to Duckus, but even Steve didn't seem to see it after the first time.

"Come here, Tigg, quick," Duckus called, using the nickname he had chosen for me from Winnie the Pooh. We had not been in the house more than thirty seconds before he was out the door. He darted to the opposite side of the huge wraparound deck and motioned for me to follow. On the walk below stood one of those icons of the masculine form—an expansive back and chest atop thick, long-boned legs all wrapped in generous layers of tanned muscle and joined tightly together at the waist. This mass of maleness was clad in a teensy-weensy yellow bikini, sexy on the beach, but more than a bit whorish on the boardwalk. This was not just a pose queen, I thought to myself. His blatant immodesty made him even more attractive to me.

"Do you want him, Tigg?" Duckus asked playfully. The Adonis had stopped and was looking up at my lover. Fully clothed, Duckus turned heads in San Francisco. Now even the gods stopped in their tracks. "Should I ask him up?"

Duckus had once embarrassed me like this before. The purpose was to show he was not at all intimidated by my rather free and open sexuality. I wasn't horny, but I didn't want to put a kibosh on what Duckus was doing either. The god did come up and turned out to be quite a gentleman—intense, educated, interesting, and careful not to be intrusive.

The following day he came over for lunch, after which we all enjoyed a fabulous romp.

No, I thought, sitting up again and brushing the beach off the back of my head, Duckus's ashes will have to stay with me in San Francisco. I wondered if the golden stud was on the island again this year. Probably, but not at tea, I thought. Not his style.

The next morning was cloudy, so I went to the gym. After a hard workout that lasted almost two hours, he showed up. Perfect! I was wet, pumped, and leaving. It took less than thirty seconds to determine that the embers we had left unstoked were not yet cold. A surge of satisfaction pulsed through my veins as I strode toward the harbor with the confidence of a prince in his own lands.

Kirk

At the grocery store I ran into Kirk, a slight, sexy man about thirty years old whom I'd met on a previous trip. Like many New Yorkers, this witty queen had played a number of roles—actor, artist, waiter, butler. After some initial niceties he lobbed one of those oblique compliments that is at once a bit rude and a bit of a come-on.

"It's always nice to see another tramp looking so well," he grinned. "Especially in 1990. What's your secret?" Our banter quickly turned toward HIV, and I realized we were starting one of those conversations that I wanted to capture on tape. He was both big on wheatgrass and insistent that the fear of death was killing people. I told him about my project, and we agreed to discuss things further the next day at noon. Meanwhile the sun was teasing us with the possibility of a beach day, and both of us were anxious to get out of the produce section.

While the next morning's news reviewed America's strategic options for waging war in the Persian Gulf, I grabbed two beach chairs and a couple of beers to reenter the war against AIDS. Should we bomb the virus or concentrate on securing the bunkers, I wondered? When Kirk arrived on the beach, we moved up near the dunes for semiprivacy, and I carefully aligned our towels slightly ahead of the sun's path. This was the first interview I had ever done on the beach. Oh, that war and work might always be so pleasant!

"Tell me when you first heard about AIDS, GRID [gay-related immun-odeficiency], HIV—whatever it was called back then," I began.

"It was after I moved to San Francisco. That's when we started hearing about a gay cancer going around and that people were suddenly going to pieces in a matter of days or weeks. That was 1982. I spent a lot of time in the city, but I lived in San Jose, where I was acting with a children's theater company. We performed there and we also toured. When my contract expired two years later, I did a few restaurants in the Bay Area as well. Then in June of 1984 I moved to New York."

"So you were just twenty-four when you first started hearing about it. What was that like?"

"It made me concerned about my own behavior patterns because that's what everybody was saying it was associated with. It wasn't being gay. It wasn't genes or anything like that. It was behavior—especially bathhouse behavior and drugs. Those were the predominant issues that seemed to keep coming into play. At least that's what I was hearing. Nobody was even talking about safe sex then, just general behavior. So it made me reflective in that sense."

"Did you feel initially that you were part of the affected group?"

"No. I felt outside of it. I felt like the average Joe Blow on the street, getting most of his information in the papers. Then I began to hear it through other people as well. You know, that's how things come to us in the larger world. You get them in the big media way—hear them, see them, read them. Then they come closer to you through other people's experiences. Finally, they touch you.

"I knew people in San Francisco who had AIDS, but they were, at best, acquaintances. My friend Anton was dealing with it when I moved to New York in 1984. Then somebody I was working with came down with it. That must have been in 1986, about the time that I tested positive. He started developing one thing after another. It was hard to see it affect him because he had a very prolonged illness with lots of really debilitating steps. That was not nice.

"By 1986 I knew that I had to be tested. I figured I would test positive, but I had to know. I'm a firm believer in truth. You got to face it, one way or the other. I don't remember what I was dealing with, but I wasn't feeling great. I went to the doctor to have a physical, and he asked if I wanted to be tested right away, and I said, 'Yes, definitely. It's time to know.'"

"So you didn't go through this business of, should I or shouldn't I take the test?"

"Yeah, a little bit, but like I said, I figured I would test positive, and therefore I should know about it. I had faced a life-threatening illness before. When I moved to San Francisco in 1982, I came down with hepatitis B. I got hit with it pretty bad. But the real problem was that, even though I was only out of commission for a month, I didn't get over it. I was chronic. I was antigen-positive and antibody-negative.

"I only learned about being chronic over the course of time, by going back for lots of visits to the doctor and having lots of blood work done. Normally, 'hep' is something that takes time to recover from, but as time went by, they decided I wasn't responding. Then they put me into a category and called me 'chronic.' I learned a lot about serious disease then. As a chronic hepatitis carrier my chances of developing liver cancer were fifty times the norm. That really freaked me out. I was scared because I realized this was serious, this could take my life, this could really do me in.

"I was still chronic when I went to see the doctor in '86 and took the HIV test, but somewhere about late 1988 my chronic hepatitis reversed. My antigen became negative, and I developed the antibody. My doctor was freaked out, but I was overjoyed! It was pretty rare. If you didn't develop the hepatitis antibody after about a year's time, they put you in the chronic group. So all of a sudden it changed, and of course what was that attributed to? I don't know. I think attitude—where your head's at—makes all the difference in the world.

"I went on a major wheatgrass thing, which I am still actively participating in. I got exposed to that in 1982. A friend of mine from Chicago was into it because he said some folks who had been experiencing AIDS symptoms went into a bit of a remission when they OD'd on this wheatgrass shit. I began drinking it on and off between 1982 and 1984. I'd drink it when I could get it, which wasn't very often. When I moved to New York, there were so many health shops and juice bars around town, it was much easier to get than it was in San Jose or even L.A. It's incredible, but health retail outlets are a lot more available in New York. So I began drinking quite a bit of it until I finally realized that I should just get my own goddamn juicer so I could have it when I wanted it. I like to drink about two to three ounces first thing in the morning. I keep it in my mouth and let the saliva work on it for a while—it's also very good for your mouth and gum tissues. It's like intense food—whoa!—major energy rush! So I attribute much of my recovery from the hep to wheatgrass.

"For a while I became a vegetarian, but then I realized that I really need meat. I really need meat—in more ways than one, of course! I've also been on a maintenance dosage of Zovirax, and I think that came into play as well. I mean, hepatitis is a virus. If you're able to curb any other viral activity or keep it at a low ebb, your body's healing process is going to be able to concentrate more in a weak area."

"So when did you start the Zovirax?"

"About the time that I tested positive, about four years ago. I had a case of hairy leukoplakia, and I've been prone to develop cold sores—herpes in my mouth—since I was a small child. I started out pretty heavy duty. Well, some people do eat quite a lot of it. He started me on about twenty capsules a day. Is that a lot?"

"Yes."

"He put me on a lot to begin with, and he cut it in half pretty shortly thereafter."

"Had you ever had genital herpes as well?"

"No. Never had it, knock on wood."

"So he just put you on that for the hep?" I asked, hoping to learn something new.

"Mostly for the hairy leukoplakia. He really didn't associate it with hepatitis. Back then they didn't know what Zovirax was going to be good for. They just knew that it seemed to have some antiviral effects and didn't seem toxic. My doctor's attitude—and consequently my own because it made sense to me—was that if it didn't seem to hurt me, why not? Also, my insurance was paying for it at the time. Now I'm supposed to take six a day. That's basically where it's at. I don't make myself crazy if I miss here and there or if I forget to take it because the hairy leuko-plakia cleared up a long time ago. I've been pretty clear of that at least for a year and a half. So that's fine by me! It cleared up right away. But if I cut back to a certain point or if I didn't take the medication at all, it would resurface.

"I had real problems resolving the fact that I might be dependent on some sort of chemical. Good, bad, or indifferent, Zovirax is a drug, a substance, and I didn't like the idea that I might have to keep that in my life all the time. I like to be able to think that our bodies can take care of themselves through their own natural means. But in certain respects HIV is like any other debilitating illness like diabetes or heart problems. They all give you a message, and you'd better fucking listen to it, or you're going to be in a bad boat. If it means you have to sustain yourself through means of some minor medication, then that's what it means.

"I was actually given an ARC diagnosis at the time, but I didn't find that out until a year later. I had some lymph nodes in the back of my neck and a few under my arms. Those cleared up with the Zovirax, too. So three symptoms gave me an ARC diagnosis: HIV positive, hairy leukoplakia, and lymphadenopathy. I don't hold much stock in the ARC diagnosis. That's just another person labeling me. Two of the three have pretty much subsided. They don't seem to be an issue. They seem to be in control. They aren't bothering me."

"You've told me that you're on Zovirax and wheatgrass. Are you doing anything else?"

"Exercising regularly is vital. I was no major jock when I was a kid, but as I've gotten older, I've become convinced that exercise is vital for human health and stability. When I say exercise, it's not just moving muscles but moving the oxygen around. The respiratory system is one of our basic life supports. What are there, five systems in the body? To thoroughly give yourself an oxygen exchange every day or every other day is vital. It means you're getting rid of all that bad air, that bad energy, and taking in the good and healthy stuff. It's the only way your blood— I mean, this thing affects the blood—it's the only way your blood will stay healthy and alive.

"I also watch my diet. Very rarely will you see me junk out. Like I said, I tried the vegetarian scene for a while, but I couldn't do it, especially in New York. This city just throws off too much energy, too much whatever. Maybe some people can do it, but I realized I needed some meat protein to keep me sort of grounded."

"So you're not doing AZT?"

"Oh, no. At the time I went to be tested in 1986, my T cells were around 750, and they stayed that way, in spite of the other things that were going on with me, until last summer. I see my doctor every three months. He's very regimented with the blood work routine, and the T cells seemed to be gradually dropping. Still, he wasn't very alarmed because the p24 wasn't getting activated and all the rest of the numbers were very healthy and seemed to be in balance.[1] So he didn't place much stock in it. Of course, that's easy for him to say. It's my T cells that were dropping."

"How far did they drop?"

"They dropped to 450, I think. That was probably in October or

November of 1989. He wasn't alarmed at all. They had just raised the level for AZT to 500, so he mentioned it in passing, but he didn't recommend it. But I wouldn't have gone on it at that point even if he had. It's never gotten to that. AZT has never been an issue for me. Three months later they jumped up 150, so I'm back over 600. That was my last trip. That would have been last November. Yes, and I'm due for another one here. I'll make an appointment next week."

"So you let it go a little longer than every three months. Sometimes nine or—"

"Well, it's because now I don't have insurance. I've been without insurance now for a year or a year and a half. I was a little concerned when the numbers were dropping and thought, maybe we have to keep a good watch on it. But when they jumped back up to 600, I thought maybe I could take an extra month or so before I do them again. Maybe I'm getting cocky already, but I really am a firm believer that you have to know as soon as possible. What you don't know can kill you."

"Do you keep track of any of the other numbers? Your ratios or percents?"

"Mostly I pay attention to my T cells. Every physical I go over my complete rundown with him, all the numbers. He doesn't like it because it takes up time. He glances over it and says they're fine or whatever, but I make him go through them all and ask how it compares to last time. My liver enzymes are still slightly elevated, and I figure that's probably due to scarring from the hepatitis, so I always ask him about those.

"My doctor is actually very interesting. I've been with him since 1986. He's a Buddhist. He's gay. He's been in a relationship for quite some time. I'd say he's in his forties, but God, his name is Wolfgang, and he's just as German as the name implies. He's a hard-assed, cynical son-of-a-bitch in many ways. It's hard to realize that this man could be a Buddhist. He's really pragmatic in terms of what he'll actually give serious attention to. He almost scoffs at anything I might have to say about wheatgrass juice.

"A good friend of mine went to a detox center in Arizona and got himself cleaned out. I asked Wolfgang once what kind of merit he would put in something like that, and he said: 'None whatsoever. If I ever wanted to leave being a doctor and make a lot of money being a charlatan, that's the sort of thing I would do.' He doesn't have much faith in anything but straight Western approaches to medicine and science. I appreciate the fact that he's very analytical and critical, but I don't listen solely to him. My God, he comes off really pessimistic. He really does."

▼ ▼ ▼

Kirk may have been the first holistic queen I'd met who didn't blast physicians for not sharing his airy-fairy beliefs. He had no interest in talking cosmic consciousness with his physician. He appreciated Wolfgang's analytical approach. Kirk's experience at the doctor's office was clearly not what Eric had described—fear in the presence of washed hands, white robes, and divination. Kirk seemed to be his own priest, his own confessor, his own counselor. He even offered his own sermons on healthy living.

I wondered what made Kirk different from those who knew they were at significant risk but who delayed testing and monitoring. Although Kirk had previous experience with a serious illness, the biggest difference seemed to be his notion of truth and his "firm belief" in facing it. Kirk offered no practical rationale for taking the test, nor did it seem overdetermined with meaning. His decision to get tested had nothing to do with taking antivirals or not taking antivirals. Kirk had to face the presence or absence of the virus in his body, not the presence or absence of a treatment plan. He had assumed he was antibody positive, but facing the possibility was not the same thing as assuming it.

In addition to "facing" things, Kirk incorporated two seemingly contradictory positions into his understanding. He adopted his physician's attitude toward the Zovirax as his own while at the same time being concerned about dependence on a chemical. He thought the body should take care of itself through its own natural means, but he also believed that serious illnesses were about "messages." Unlike Jason or Eric, who thought many of the messages about HIV and AIDS should be resisted in one way or another, Kirk thought serious illnesses were always personal messages to which we have to pay special attention. Even his hesitation about dependence on pills was suspended in favor of his notion that illness and loss are meant to teach us something, to be transformative. I wondered whether Kirk's position on facing death was primarily philosophical or experiential and asked if he had ever lost anyone really close to him.

▼ ▼ ▼

"I lost my best friend, Anton. I met him in 1978 when I went to college—the first week. We lived together for three years in college, before I moved to California. When I moved to New York in 1987, we lived together again. Of course, we had stayed very close during all that time anyway. He died in 1988. It happened very quick, which I was very grateful for. He came back from a Christmas vacation with a cold and a cough and was worried that it might be pneumonia, but the doctor said it wasn't. From Christmas to late March, he didn't feel great. He was working through a lot of shit and thought he was feeling physical manifestations of his emotional work. He wasn't sure.

"It pretty much happened in about a week. We were both very busy. I was leaving the house early and getting back late. We weren't seeing much of each other. Living in New York, you can go days without seeing your roommate. He wasn't feeling great, so he had been staying home from work. I wasn't sure what was going on because he'd be in bed when I left and when I got back home. We'd maybe just exchange a few words over the phone. After a week I had an evening off. I think it was a Thursday night. When I saw him, I thought, my God, he's a basket case! He had gotten weak. He had severe diarrhea. He wasn't eating. I mean, all of a sudden I took a good look at him and saw that physically he had deteriorated in this week to an alarming point.

"We were both very worried, and he was all freaked out, so we called the hotline. A scenario was beginning to brew in his mind. I don't know how rational he was at the time. I think he was getting very fearful. We talked a lot. I had to go out and buy him diapers because he had diarrhea so bad that he didn't make it to the toilet, and then he didn't have any energy to clean it up, and, oh God, that was only half a day. The next afternoon I took him to the hospital.

"They admitted him. He had pneumonia. Anton had never taken the test. After a couple days they put him on a respirator to make him breathe easier. Then he started fighting it, so then they sedated him. A day or two later a lung collapsed, so they sedated him further and he became even more dependent on the respirator. It all lasted about five or six weeks from the time he was admitted until he died. Most of the time he was so heavily sedated to keep him from fighting the machine or whatnot that he wasn't able to communicate.

"It was very, very hard on me to see somebody—he was sedated. He bloated up like Elvis. We joked with him. Then he went back down. It got to the point where he was developing bedsores. It was just hard to see. He wasn't in a coma, but it was like he was in a coma. For the first two weeks maybe you'd get small signs out of him. A tear. He'd move a finger. His eye would move, you know, signaling that he knew you were there or he knew what was going on around him.

"His family came right away. Then he seemed to go nowhere. He wasn't getting better or worse. All his friends decided he was probably waiting for his father, because his father hadn't been to see him yet. His mother, brother, and sister had. His father had suffered two strokes, so getting around and traveling were difficult. But really, Anton was the baby in the family, and his father just didn't want to see it.

"Shit. I had a number of difficult phone conversations with Anton's father, Roger. He kept saying he couldn't come, that he did not want to see him like this, that he wanted to remember him the way he was at Christmas, and if he died, so be it, but that's how he wanted to remember him. I don't get angry very often or very deeply, but that was one of the most angry moments of my life. Two or three days went by, and I called him again and he finally relented and came to see him. It was very difficult, but very essential for Roger, and very essential for Anton, I think, because about a week after Roger left to go back to St. Louis, Anton died.

"We had been playing Louise Hay tapes and told the nurses to just keep them rolling, because when you are in a coma or in a drug-conked state, you can still hear. So we tried to fill him with lots of messages. I sat with him for about two hours and—straight out of *Longtime Companion*—just basically said, 'Look, I think it's selfish for me to think that you have to stay on, and if you feel that there's a larger light for you, then let go.' It was probably the most difficult emotional moment of my life. The nurses kept coming in to see if I was okay. He died that night. I think it's self-inflating to think that he was waiting for me to say anything, but maybe he was.

"The next day I got a call from his brother, and as soon as I heard who it was, I knew. At first it was sort of numbing. I don't think I've ever felt that much physical pain. It was complete total pain, physical, emotional. It felt like my guts had been ripped out. It felt like there was an enormous hole in me.

"Everybody thought Anton and I were lovers. He had come home and met my family several times. They all thought we were lovers. A lot of acquaintances assumed that we were lovers because we were so close. But we only slept together once, and that was with a third, somebody I picked up when Anton and I were traveling on a vacation together, and Anton hopped in bed with us. It was sort of harmless, playful fun. Our relationship never took on a physical expression. We weren't ever very attracted to each other.

"He died in 1988, about a week after my birthday, late June. For a while you never know what will set you off. The tears just come out, you know. Time makes a big difference for a lot of things, but grief never goes away. There's a deep emotional wealth in having shared Anton's death. It enriched my life. I'm sorry to say that I lost an enriching part of my life because of it, but life is give and take. I don't think any of us grow unless we can learn from whatever we experience. If you just look at loss in a bad light, you're never going to get anywhere as a human being. You just aren't going to develop. You're going to be stuck in some quagmire of ego-inflated neuroses. Unless you're able to take any issue, no matter how painful, and find a good side to it, you're going to be in tough shape."

"Do you get to talk to many people about this stuff? About AIDS?"

"I'm a registered client of the GMHC. I really don't use their services because, fortunately, I haven't needed them. One of their people just called me the other day, just called to check up. I told them, 'I am very grateful that you do this, but I'm happy to say that I seem to be pretty stable and feel great and relatively happy, and the reason I registered with you was because I did have an ARC diagnosis, which doesn't hold much value for me, but somebody labeled me with it, so I'm going to take advantage of it.'

"A lot of people would say it's a disadvantage to have a label like that. Well, yes, it is, but you can also use it to your advantage as well. I registered with the GMHC so that if all of a sudden something happened, I could turn to them and maybe they could help me out. Right now all I need from the GMHC is to know that they're there if I need them. I want to continue getting the newsletter and everything. Outside of that, I don't work with any sort of support group or anything like that. I practice yoga pretty regularly. I have since I was in California in 1982. I do some meditation."

"What about your family?"

"That's a big issue for me. I was just visiting. Where to start?"

"Who are they?"

"I'm the oldest of five children. Mom and Dad are still alive. They're all in Wisconsin."

"Do they know you're gay?"

"They know I'm gay. I have another gay relative in the family, an older cousin with a lover. We do Christmas with them. They're very out within the family. It's very accepted. They're a little older. My being gay didn't become an issue until Anton became ill.

"I moved out of the house when I was fifteen. I finished high school away and then moved to college, which was a twelve-hour drive away, and then to California. So I've seen my family maybe once or twice a year since I went to college in 1978. When I've been with them, being gay hasn't ever been an issue. First, I guess, I had problems talking about it. When I did become more accepting of it, it just didn't seem important when I spent time with them. If they'd asked me, I would have gladly told them, but it didn't seem like it was important for me to bring it up, and they didn't ask.

"Then Anton got sick, and they knew that we were very close. When I told Mom he was sick and how serious it was, she broke over the phone. I told her right then, 'Look, Mom. Anton and I are friends. We have never been lovers. Yes, I'm gay, but we are not lovers. We've never slept together. If I'm at any risk, it's in no way associated with my relationship with Anton.'"

"So did you tell her at the same time you were HIV positive?"

"No. That's the big issue in my life right now. When I go to see my family, I share in their lives. My brother is married with two children. They all have the normal young lives—careers, boyfriends, wives, children. None of my family has come to see me in New York. None of them ever came to see me in San Francisco. What they know of my life they know from phone conversations, and through my cousin Christina, who is closer to me than any of my brothers and sisters. She has come to New York many times. So they know of my life through Christina, but basically they don't know much. They don't seem to have any interest. I think there's some concern, but there's some fear involved.

"This last trip home I really wanted to bring it to a head with one of my sisters. If any of them asked me, I would tell them. Why I don't volunteer it is because I don't think they'd understand it—especially my mom and dad. Their perceptions are going to be warped by what the media told them five years ago, that it's a death sentence. They would probably freak out and go buy my cemetery plot if I told them. Maybe they need to so they can come to accept it before—it's a real issue for me. I feel like I'm very open with my family. We're all very close. But there's this one thing about my life that's not getting communicated. It's not so much that I'm not communicating. With family members there's an understanding, you know. You were raised together. You know where your heads are at. You know where you're coming from. You have the same points of reference. But they don't understand this particular point of reference in my life, and it could be the overwhelming reference point in my life, certainly a major one."

▼▼▼

As a gay man with HIV, Kirk's experience with his parents is not at all unusual. Even though he had an "out" cousin and being gay was "accepted," Kirk didn't feel compelled to share that part of himself with his family until Anton got sick. Everyone knew, of course, but although the family was "close," the substance and structure of their relationships were such that Kirk never brought it up. Perhaps Kirk's initial reluctance to talk about his homosexuality helped establish silence as the norm. It would be mistaken, however, to understand Kirk's initial problem with talking about being gay as a personal, rather than a family, social, or cultural, issue. Kirk could share in his family's lives, but they couldn't share in his. Some of the closeness that Kirk felt to his family is probably romanticized, a personal adaptation to a widespread sociocultural problem.

Those who managed to resist the overwhelmingly negative construction of HIV leading invariably to AIDS were often not eager to broach the topic with loved ones. Even though men with HIV often lived much longer than women with breast cancer, there was almost no hope discourse around HIV/AIDS. Those like Michael Callen who dared to talk about surviving AIDS were warned that it was bad for fundraising, bad for "AIDS, Inc." Even Nathan, a psychiatrist, armed himself with a videotape on hope and self-healing before approaching his family. Having to care for a family member's reaction proved to be too much for many of the men I knew. The burden was often easier to carry alone.

I switched topics and asked what sex and drugs had been like since testing positive.

▼▼▼

"I don't necessarily put sex and drugs together, by no means. Let's deal with drugs first because that's much more cut-and-dry. I appreciate them. I value the altered experience. Everybody has addictive tendencies. I do as well, but I seem to be able to control them a little better than some people I know. I believe anything is okay in moderation. My sense of moderation has become much more moderate than it used to be, and if I want to use any substances, as I do every so often, I make sure that I supplement myself with lots of vitamins and sleep. And I eat. I believe that drugs can wear your body down, but they don't have to if you take a little bit of care. You know, you have a cold and your body deals with it by telling you to sleep. So you sleep and you get over it. The same with drugs. You don't push yourself. I don't understand these people who do one drug after the next and go for a weekend without sleep. I could do it maybe when I was twenty, but I don't know how they do it."

"So how much?"

"What sort of quantity? Well, I don't buy marijuana any longer because that is the one drug that, if I have it, I'll smoke it, even if it's just one hit a day. And if I smoke every day, it begins to have an effect on me. I'll share a joint now and again, and that's fine because I'm not going to have it the next day, but I will not buy it. I don't do speed anymore. I don't do cocaine. I never bought it or did much of it in the first place. I do Ecstasy now and again. I did some mushrooms not too long ago, which I like a lot, but you can't get them very often. How often do I do it? Once every six weeks, maybe four. Summertime is more, undoubtedly, and that's fine."

"Do you ever have any conflict with yourself over shoulds and shouldn'ts?'"

"Well, that's just feeling guilt over something. Do something and then give yourself shit about it? Well, goddamnit, if you're going to do it, then do it and enjoy it and get over it. Accept it. I do like the experience, the altered state, the high."

"So it's resolved for you? It's not a source of conflict?"

"I'll tell you why. As I do drugs now, as I enjoy them, they don't seem to be affecting my health, at least not in a manner that I can see. Long term, who knows? I would stop using whatever I do use if I began to see something happening. You know, some things go downhill. When some people I know begin to get sick, they double whatever they're doing. They have a death wish. I don't. So I can say right now that I don't have a conflict with it. Well, I was raised in the Midwest as a Roman Catholic, so deep down there's some inherent, learned guilty voice that does come up now and again and says, 'You dumb-ass.' But I've learned to address that voice pretty well. It's really unnecessary to put myself through all of that. In my opinion, if you're going to do something, then do it full out. Commitment is a major word in my life and my experience. If you want to do something, then commit yourself fully to it. Try not to do something half-assed."

"I'm real interested in what the death wish thing is about. Do you have any of it?"

"A death wish?"

"You said you didn't, but talk about that a little."

"I used to be a major party animal, and I used to be able to really carry on in college. When I first came out, I could be ridiculous. I used to think that some sort of death wish was behind some of my behavior. Maybe it was. I don't associate a death wish with any of my drug behaviors now. They are about living. Maybe I'm kidding myself, but when it comes to a death wish, I can only talk about how I see it exhibited in other people. Am I being self-deceiving in saying that there's none in myself? I don't know. There could be some in everybody, but there's not much of one in me. I'm a pretty firm believer and practitioner of life, of living. The reason I think I can say that is because I recognize that death is a vital part of life."

"Does the death wish you see in other people bother you?"

"Yes. I saw one person recently who really did it to himself. He was so fucked up every time I saw him. He knew he was sick and just took the 'I'm just dancing till I drop' attitude. And he recently did. I try not to judge it. He was doing whatever he had to do, learning in whatever way he had to. It all becomes a question of how much empathy can you have? How much can you relate? I don't identify much with it. It would be interesting to explore the death wish as an actor."

"What about your sex life? How has that been affected?"

"Well, I've learned to take the cold shower. I was complete trash before I took the test. I mean, I knew I would test positive. I was a bathhouse babe. When I kicked down that fucking repressive midwestern door, I did it full-heartedly, with firm commitment. And I was trash in college. Being a performance arts major, I had plenty of time to do that!

"I was in Chicago a lot, and even when I first went to San Francisco, I was doing the bathhouse scene. I curtailed that very quickly when I began to hear that people suspected all those anonymous contacts had a lot to do with contracting 'the cancer.' If anything, I've come to realize that as much as I like sex, and as much as I realize sex can take me from myself and at the same time take me within myself like nothing else I've had, it's not the be-all and end-all. Sex is about a spiritual and emotional sharing between two people, not just a physical sharing. It's too easy to look at sex from just the physical side."

"So for you, it's been problematic, not problematic?"

"I went through different stages. For two years I didn't touch another man. No sex at all. Months went by and I was beginning to go crazy, but after a year it hardly crossed my mind. I don't even remember how it happened again. Sex is that thing—you get some poontang once, and you want more in another hour. I've never had a boyfriend. I've never been in love. I've never dated anybody longer than six months. I have not yet in my life connected sex with a deep emotional commitment with any other person. It's always been pretty much a date, a one-night stand or whatever. I still believe firmly in it, though. I've been practicing safe sex for as long as I found out I was positive, so I do not feel guilty about how I behave in sex."

"And what do you mean by safe sex?"

"I've terminated pretty much in the very broadest sense the exchange of fluids. I'll go down on somebody, as long as there's no exchange."

"You mean as long as they don't cum in your mouth?"

"Right."

"What about fucking?"

"Well, nobody really gets near me without a rubber. It just comes down to that. I would say that in the last three years maybe somebody's got it in me, and it's in there for ten seconds, and I say, 'Okay, enough practice, now comes the real thing.' It's just not worth the chance or risk. So that's basically the way I define it in terms of affecting my behavior. Hey, anything else goes!

"If anything, I've found that safe sex has enriched my sexual expression. No doubt of it. Learn to use your imagination and your mind more. It's definitely made me much more aware of the level of pain and pleasure and more willing to explore those boundaries."

"You've gotten more into S&M?"

"Not really. I certainly wouldn't call it any sort of hard-core."

"Light S&M?"

"Light S&M! Sounds like a radio station! Rough trade, babe. How else has it affected sex? That's it. But if anything, I'd say it hasn't affected sex so much as how we meet other men now. That instant, one-minute pickup just doesn't happen."

"Not even in New York?"

"On the street? No. The way it used to be, in San Francisco and Chicago, was if you were awake, you were cruising. Whatever you were doing, you were working it. Maybe it's getting older; I don't know. It's sort of like there's a time and a place.

"I think it's made other people more uptight about sex than it has myself. I recently started seeing this guy, Leonard, a very attractive man I met through my friend who goes to the detox center in Arizona—he's back there right now having his spark plugs changed. Leonard was just out of an eleven-year relationship, and they didn't practice safe sex since they were very monogamous. Or so they said, in spite of the fact that they both tested positive—so what does that say? I was really attracted to Leonard, but he was not comfortable at all with safe sex. He hadn't ever practiced it. He didn't know how. He was a real intense case, but I see that sort of behavior and those attitudes reflected in a lot of other people, too. I think the inability to deal with safe sex is really about fear, fear of death, mostly. The fear of death is paralyzing people, and not just gay men, but people in general.

"You know what HIV has really come to mean in my life? A narc faces certain risks in his line of work. So does a fireman and a window washer. So does someone with diabetes or high blood pressure. An HIV-positive person does as well. They're all just signposts to remind you to accept the fact that you will go."

A number of Kirk's ideas about life and health were similar to Jason's. Both of them believed that the attitudes one takes toward serious illness are vitally important. Both of them believed in the importance of diet, exercise, and meditation. Both of them understood that Western medicine did not have all the answers. However, when it came to thinking about HIV and death, there were huge differences. Jason was afraid to put the idea that he might die "into existence," whereas Kirk understood that death was in existence already. Kirk saw HIV as a sign to keep him from forgetting his essential nature as a mortal being. At the same time, Kirk appreciated the need for hope, and he was just as frustrated as many of the other participants in this project at the hopelessness diatribe from the experts.

"Do you want to know what really twists my panties in a bunch? The attitude that testing positive was a death sentence. That attitude pervaded the press when the HIV antibody was discovered. I don't know who might have given them that idea, but people grabbed hold of it big time! My God, it was a sea of unknowns for everybody when it came to AIDS and a time when people would grab anything. All those so-called experts were saying, 'Now there's an antibody, and it means you were exposed, and it means you're going to get AIDS, and it means you're going to die!' That really bothers me, and I think it's plenty clear now that was never the case. And I believed them at the time as well. Now that I've been on a stable course for at least four years, I've come to trust my own observations and my own experience more than the experts. They've been testing since '85, right? I know somebody who was in the initial stages in San Francisco when they began testing, and he's been positive for five or six years and he's doing great."

"And then there are people who have been positive since 1978, for twelve years already, from the old hepatitis study."

"Yes, that's right. And recently they even found some English sailor. They dug his bones up and checked him out and in 1968 this guy had an HIV antibody. So it's been around a long time. Where has it been lurking?"

"Well, I haven't heard about that one, but I've never yet been to an AIDS conference where some bimbo with a couple of graduate degrees didn't pronounce from the podium that HIV was 100 percent fatal. The doomsday sentimentality that passes for thinking on the AIDS conference circuit is about as sophisticated as the daytime soaps."

"Yeah. Back to the kitchen, bitches."

"Oh, it's not just the ladies. The gentlemen are no better. They're worse, in fact. They pontificate with a greater air of scientific authority."

"Like I said. Back to the kitchen, bitches. Or the barn if it suits you better. Just get off my dress! But the other thing that really bothers me about HIV is that it is inhibiting a lot of people. It's making them feel guilty about sex. People are just screwing their heads over with it. Didn't the sexual revolution push us forward at all? If AIDS is just going to throw us back into that Victorian-Eisenhower repression that gays and straights threw off in the sixties and seventies, what was our sexual revolution all about? That was an invaluable experience. If we can't learn from that! I wouldn't trade a night in the bathhouse for anything! And

I feel compassion for these guys who are twenty and are coming out, and they never get to spend a night in a bathhouse and fuck around with eight people in one night. I mean, that's letting your libido go crazy. That's letting your fantasy run wild. It was great to have that experience.

"As I've said, the physical act of sex is not the most important part of relationships. The most important part of relationships is the bonds that you form, the emotional, the spiritual, the intellectual bonds that you form. Those are the true values of relationships. I don't want to demean the sexual, because I think that's a valid and important means for exploring relationships and deepening them and communicating within them, but that's not where the deepest values lie. To respond to nothing but your senses and perceptions, that's strong black magic, that is voodoo, and it can really blind you to things. Maybe it's taken something like this virus to make us wake up and realize, hey look, sex is all well and good, and it's a natural expression and a form of communication and being, but it is not the most important.

"So we'd better learn from this. We have to look at HIV as an education, a signpost. It means learn from where we've been, learn from where we're at. Watch yourself. Listen to yourself. Listen to your body. Take care of yourself.

"And if it happens, it happens. Death is going to happen. The big 'D.' Get used to it. It's a part of life. From the moment you're born, you're dying. That's Buddhism, baby. That's the great wheel of suffering. Everything is transient, and you're no exception to the rule. If your ego gets involved and starts pulling some trip that you're going to survive in this world forever, you're in a sorry way."

"Nobody," I said, "gets off this island alive, boys."

▼▼▼

If anyone had a chance of making it, I thought, it would be Kirk. He wasn't afraid of death or doctors. He wasn't filled with anger, shame, or guilt. He was happy with who he was. He wouldn't ever "just say no," but he knew when to stop. He wasn't afraid of sex, but he knew when to take the proverbial cold shower. He wasn't in love, but the world was full of infinite possibility for him. Wheatgrass was powerful, and so was oxygen, but he didn't get neurotic and try to do every possible holistic or allopathic treatment.

After we finished talking, I shut off the tape, ripped off my bathing suit, and ran for the water. The mixture of sweat, sand, and suntan oil that had baked itself into a nasty crust disintegrated on impact. In an instant the Atlantic's chilling embrace restored a sense of wholesome innocence. After five minutes of bobbing up and down in the strong swells, my body yearned again for the slow bake of the island sun.

Kirk was packed up and ready to go. I wondered what my friends Eric and Jason would think of him. "See you at tea?" he asked.

"Absolutely."

I carefully shook the sand from my towel, realigned it with the sun, and, without protection, offered the falling shafts, beams, and ultraviolet rays unrestricted access to my still-dripping body. "Walk the edge, sweetheart," whispered some spirit from the sands. "This is heaven."

Damian

After a long glorious day in the sun, I was up for "tea." A quick shower, a fresh black tank top, a carefully selected pair of my favorite nondescript shorts, and I was ready. I crossed over to the bay side and walked down to the harbor to tea, ordered an Absolut gimlet, and surveyed the largely preppy crowd. One guy stood out for me—tall, dark, good-looking, but not traditionally handsome. He eschewed the standard Top-Siders for a pair of black high-top tennis shoes. These, together with his ripped, way-too-short cutoffs, forced the eye up and down his brown lanky legs to excellent effect. We caught each other's eye but didn't speak. Maybe later.

We did meet later, at the disco. His name was Damian. Fire bells woke us the next morning. He pulled on his high-tops, slipped into his cutoffs, and went out to investigate. "Not the condos," he reported. "You're safe. I'm going to get out of here and do some wash. Want me to make some coffee first?"

"Sure," I sighed, and rolled over to watch him grind the beans. I liked him. A Long Island boy, he'd been hearing about AIDS since 1983, two years after having moved to New York City. He didn't take big note of it at the time, assuming it was affecting only debilitated, drug-addicted homosexuals. Since both of us had assumed that the other was probably positive, we didn't even mention HIV until that morning after. He was a graduate student in social work and showed some interest in my project. We agreed to postpone talking about HIV until we felt more up to an in-depth conversation. He invited me over to do some laundry of my own later in the day. After a workout and some lazy hours reading, I tossed the tape recorder in with my dirty clothes and headed down Ocean Walk.

"I wondered if you'd actually make it today," called a voice from inside the house. "I'm going to make margaritas. Want one?"

We settled into a couple of chaise lounges on the deck and absorbed the tequila-tinged light. There was just enough sun to translate a vague threat of rain into a sticky, sexy humidity. Every visible house was painted in shades of gray that blended with beach and boardwalk. A few weathered ones peeled, but even those glowed like sterling roses. Shabby here and there, but it all fit. The whole place was decadent, expensive, perverse. Like England, I mused, past her prime, buggered beyond belief, yet somehow still elegant, still interesting. How was it that gay men could find themselves in such intimate situations so quickly, so easily? I really didn't even know this guy, and here we were, soaking it all in. It took a few minutes of silence before we found that our mood was more talkative than sexual, and I flipped on the recorder.

"Where did you first hear about it?" I asked.

"Probably in the *Times*. Then I picked up some of the gay newspapers to get a better perspective on what was happening in the community. That was about '83. I had just been out a couple of years then—well, not out really. That's just when I started having sex with men. So I was still fighting a lot of my own issues and coming to terms with being homosexual—and just beginning to let my family and friends know. I wasn't completely entrenched in the whole homosexual world yet."

"When did you get tested?"

"About three years ago, in spring of 1987. I'd just gotten a private doctor who told me that I had some slightly swollen glands and that my T cells were low [250]. He suggested I get tested for my own knowledge. He suspected that I probably was HIV positive anyway, but thought it would be a good idea to know for sure."

"So you suspected that you were?"

"I was pretty certain I was at that point. I really didn't even need to be tested. I'd had a lot of contact, and I knew enough people who were getting sick and testing positive. By that time I had more knowledge of how widespread this thing was. It would have surprised me if I had escaped."

"Were there any reasons why you didn't get the test done before 1987?"

"I guess I was afraid to have it finalized. I wasn't sure how I would react to absolutely finding out. There was no out at that point. There was nothing positive to do to save yourself. You were just helpless. I assumed I was positive anyway, so it didn't seem to be a real necessity at the time. It wasn't going to tell me anything that I didn't know already. Plus I don't like going to doctors. I don't like technicians. I can't stand the whole atmosphere. I didn't want to be in a situation where I'd have this huge, strong emotional reaction and then have some idiot who's being very distant and objective, standing there telling me this incredibly horrible news. I didn't want to fall apart and have no one to lean on. I wanted to be secure with a doctor. I'd wanted to have a doctor I was comfortable with, someone who would help me through if something happened."

"What was it like then to get the results from the doctor?"

"Oh God, I was crying. But I have a pretty incredible doctor, so I was lucky in the way it was presented to me. It was hard, but I wasn't crushed. He was very kind and very sensitive to what was going on, and he was very positive in a lot of respects. He suggested what I could do at that time, which wasn't much, but he also did the best he could to let me know statistically there was no way of knowing, that it was not a death sentence."

"So even though you assumed you were positive, and even though the results were delivered in a good way, there was still a lot of emotion attached to it."

"Yeah. I was sort of surprised. I really didn't expect to get the rush of emotion that I got. But I had to. You can't come face-to-face with the possibility of your death in a few years and not have emotion. As much as I went around thinking that I was positive anyway, there's a difference between thinking you're positive and dealing with your death. Until I really heard I was positive, the reality hadn't really set in."

Damian did not say he thought he was positive because his T cells were low or because he had swollen lymph nodes or even because his doctor thought he probably was. He thought he was positive because he had "had a lot of contact" and knew "how widespread this thing was." Like many other gay men, Damian's referent point was not what was going on in his own body, but who he was in relation to the rest of his world.

Damian had also predicted that his intellectual assumption about being HIV positive would not prevent him from having an emotional response once that status was empirically confirmed. My own story had been very different. I went to the anonymous test site because my lover, Duckus, had insisted that we both get tested. I also assumed I was positive but neither expected nor experienced much of an emotional response. I thought that confirmation of being HIV positive might provide greater motivation for the holistic practices I thought I should be doing. That was in 1985, when—unlike later on—I was hearing that only 20 percent of those who tested positive would come down with AIDS. Another factor that made my story different from Damian's was that my ex-lover, Steve, was already seriously ill. Perhaps I was too consumed with my own grief to worry about what might happen to me at some future point. The present was too full of its own difficulties.

However, Damian's experience with receiving his HIV test results was very different from Nathan's, Ron's, and my own. Nathan's physician loaded his first T-cell count of 200 with frightful meanings by asking him if he was sitting down before announcing the results over the phone. Luke's test counselor and support group were incredibly "heavy" about an HIV-positive test result. All of those tests took place fairly early in the history of AIDS at a time when we really didn't know what they meant. Damian's physician was both honest and professional enough to admit that "statistically there was no way of knowing," a very different message from the one received by many people with HIV.

"Sometimes I think dealing with my own death, even going through the horrible death that it is, wouldn't be as hard as having to watch my family go through it. They've been absolutely fantastic. They've all rallied around. The whole thing has completely changed my life and my relationship with them. I got a different perspective. Family issues and career goals became much more immediate for me. Lots of things came right into my face. It's been very lucky in a weird way. I've made changes in my life that, Jesus, I don't know how long it would have taken me to make.

"I finally got my act together to go back to school. I was having a very hard time getting serious about what I was doing. I'd been working in social services since I was fifteen years old, and I just wouldn't get myself back in school. I kept avoiding it. Now I'm back into school and I'm working on my career goals."

"That's incredible," I replied. "Most people in their twenties who find out they're positive have a lot of trouble dealing with career goals. But you went into a two-year program that includes summer school to prepare for a future that is questionable."

"Well, in the beginning I thought I was going to die and I was very depressed. I was going out more; I was drinking and drugging more. I had just thought, to hell with it. I'm going to get it. I'm going to die and that's it. That went on for maybe six months, and then I realized that it wasn't going to get me; I was going to get myself. I was just beating myself up—basically trying to kill myself. So I just picked up my stuff and went home."

"Did you think maybe you'd live for a while? Or was it because it didn't matter whether you lived for a while or not—you still needed to do something?"

"It was more like the latter. I don't know that I'm going to live for a while. There's no way for me to know it. I figured that I had to just continue and figure out what I wanted to do, what was important to me. When I looked at my life, I realized that what was important to me was the kind of work I'd been doing. I knew I wasn't anywhere near my potential. It's funny. The guy who was my roommate at this internship got lymphoma in February and died in three months. He was in the last year of his master's program.

"It was an incredible blow to the whole group of us who were in this internship. They graduated him in the ceremony and everything. That was my biggest fear in some ways, to do all this work and then drop dead. It's been very difficult for me. I fought off going back to school because I don't like school. I've never felt comfortable in the academic world, for some reason. I've been surprised at how well I've done this time around, but it's been very hard on me. To go through all this hell, and then die in the last few months! I don't know. I just told myself that I couldn't look at it that way. I have to be much more day-to-day about things, regardless of whether I get this degree or not. My own personal growth and learning has ultimately been more important. And I've been impressed by myself for getting through and doing as well as I have."

"God, that sounds big. Big stuff."

"Real big. I'm sure I would never be where I am today if it hadn't of been for this disease. I probably wouldn't have gone back to school. Professionalizing myself is just an outcome of a place I've come to internally. It has more to do with how I've grown emotionally and spiritually than anything else. That's probably been the biggest benefit of this disease."

"Kind of an inward growing up?"

"Absolutely."

"So do you feel like you're one of those cancer patients who says in some ways my cancer was a gift?"

"In a funny way, yes. I hate to say it, but yeah. It's absolutely true. If I didn't have to pick myself up after crashing when I finally did start to deal with HIV, I'm sure that nothing would have changed for quite some time. I also felt on an unconscious level that my survival was at stake. If I was ever going to be an autonomous person again and take care of myself, I had to get a degree. I couldn't function any longer on the kind of salaries and limited opportunity I had before. So it meant an awful lot to me.

"In any case, things have picked up since then, and I've calmed down—especially since the summer—and I'm feeling much more relaxed and in control of the school situation."

▼ ▼ ▼

"Did you make any changes, any sexual changes?"

"Well, I was with my lover at the time, and we started using rubbers."

"And that was not problematic?"

"Problematic between us?"

"Yeah. Was it easy to do?"

"No, it wasn't easy to do at all. It was horrible. I didn't want to use them. I didn't like them. I don't like the way they feel. It's been hard, you know, because I was used to a certain type of sex. My whole concept of sexuality had to change. I had to find other ways of enjoying sex without it always being flesh on flesh. There's a certain amount of intimacy that seems to diminish when you use rubbers, and it can be difficult to keep the sexual arousal going with them. When you're with one person and you make a commitment to doing it, you just do it. After we broke up, and I had multiple partners at different times, it was more difficult to always insist on them, to always bring it up. Once I'm heated up and having an initial contact with somebody, I find it more difficult."

"So your experience goes against the published research that says people in relationships are having the hardest time using rubbers and those who are outside of relationships find it easier. That's not true in your experience?"

"Not true in my case."

"Do you go through, like, any rationalizations, or is it just really the heat of the moment?"

"Well, I mean, rationalizations, sure, to some degree. The medical community is so iffy about what's going on—whether more contact is really detrimental for someone who is already HIV positive. Nobody has ever cum in me in years and years."

"So we're talking about fucking without rubbers, but not to the point of ejaculation?"

"Definitely not."

"Do you feel like you're putting yourself significantly more at risk when you fuck without rubbers?"

"I don't know how to determine that. There doesn't seem to be any absolute determination of whether you are or you aren't. Sometimes I feel like maybe I am. I guess that's why I do it, because I don't know for sure, and there is nothing that comes close to that kind of feeling. Having good sex is one of the few things that I find pleasurable in life. It's just a very difficult thing to say no to. There are so many questions about what is or what isn't safe, and I can hypothesize as much as I like. I can forbid myself certain things and then be run down on the street the next day and not die from this thing at all. I don't know about being that disciplined. I have enough guilt and anxiety. Most of the time I certainly don't have risky sex. It depends on the person I happen to be with and what the energy is between us. It doesn't always even come to that question. I don't always have that kind of intimate sex, not at all."

"So are you fairly satisfied with these changes you've made?"

"No, I'm not completely satisfied. I'd love to be perfect at everything. I'd love to be completely disciplined in every aspect of my life. This is just another part of the whole scheme of things. I'm not perfect. I'm not completely disciplined. This is just another area where I'm not. I know we're talking life and death, but we're also talking a lot of vagueness."

▼ ▼ ▼

Many of the men I know decided to clean up their acts after learning that they were HIV positive, perhaps responding to the San Francisco AIDS Foundation's "Be Here for the Cure" posters. Damian didn't exactly fit into that group, however. He actually did more drugs and alcohol after testing positive. When he started cleaning up his act and focusing on larger issues, such as family and career, he did so both because of and in spite of HIV.

Damian did say that he probably wouldn't have gone back to school had it not been for HIV. However, he didn't change his life around as a result of an infusion of hope or positive thinking. He didn't turn his life around as part of a goal to live longer. Damian's story was not in any way focused on reducing risks.[2] Sex was one of his few great pleasures, and even though he integrated condoms into a sexual relationship, he was not convinced that it actually made any difference. The fear of reexposure was largely a theoretical danger, and Damian knew it. Damian also knew that life was full of questions about what was safe and what wasn't. He'd love to be perfect, but he questioned the wisdom of living a strict and disciplined life and seemed to simply choose life instead. Damian seemed to take his cue from people like Queen Margrethe of Denmark, who continues to enjoy her cigarettes. Even though some public health officials think the queen is a negative role model in that respect, the queen insists she is sending quite another public health message: enjoy life.

Damian also had a different relationship with his family than did many of the other men in this study. Unlike Kirk, who thought his family would become a burden if they learned of his HIV status, Damian reported that his family was fantastic. Several years earlier Damian's sister had died of cancer. So unlike many families of young gay men, Damian's had had previous experience with loss, and that may have helped them cope with his HIV status.

▼▼▼

"Okay. So you were positive, your T cells were 250, and at that time they weren't putting people on AZT.

"Actually, I did go on some medication for a while. I went on some—I don't remember the name of it right now. That stuff they give heroin addicts."

"Not methadone. Naltrexone?"

"Yes."

"Which seemed like a completely innocuous thing to do?"

"Right. I knew it was innocuous. I knew it wouldn't be debilitating. People have maintained on it for like twenty years or something without any effects."

"Yeah. I've forgotten the theory behind that, but I remember it was attractive."

"Yeah. It was supposed to help pull your T cells up.

"Did it?"

"No. I was on it for less than a year. I had started it in November 1988, and my T cells didn't seem to go anywhere. Then I had an infection last summer, a fistula that had to be removed surgically. That freaked me out. I had never experienced anything that I couldn't spontaneously rid myself of basically. It really scared me. Anyway, I went off the stuff before the surgery."

"Oh, right. Otherwise the pain meds wouldn't have worked!"

"Yeah, and that would have been hell! So I went off it then, and then I really cleaned up my act after that. I wasn't drinking or smoking or doing anything. I was working out and running and taking care of myself—more stringently than I had ever done in my life, and in a very disciplined way, for two months or so. Then I went back on the stuff about two weeks before going to get tested again, and my T cells had gone up to over 500."

"So how long were you off the naltrexone?"

"Oh, something like six or eight weeks. I didn't attribute it to the naltrexone."

"Your T cells were up to 500, and you didn't attribute it to the naltrexone?"

"No, because I had been off it for eight weeks and only back on it for two. I'd never had a change in my T cells when I was on it before. Only very slight changes. At that point I began to think that this had more to do with taking care of myself and less to do with taking that stuff. So I stopped taking it."

"Then what? Since last summer you've been in school, taking care of yourself, and not doing drugs?"

"No, I haven't been that great about drugs, to be honest with you. I've been off and on, but nothing like years ago. I have been drinking some."

"So less than before, but still more than you were doing when you had the fistula?"

"Yeah. This past February I was retested and was in the high 300s. So it's gone down. My physician suggested AZT, but I told him I didn't want to go on it at that point, that I wanted to wait it out and be tested a few more times. I haven't been back yet, but I'm going in a couple of weeks. He feels I'm borderline and said he'd be willing to go either way with me right now because of where I've been over all these years."

"So what do you think of AZT? Are you familiar with the research that came out in September of last year?"

"Yeah, I read it. But I'm not comfortable being on something as strong as AZT. It seems to be fairly debilitating over an extended period of time. It's a big issue for me. I certainly will go on it at some point. I'm not completely averse to it anymore. In the beginning people were getting as sick from the AZT as they were from the illness, and I couldn't quite understand the point. I don't know. If I stay in the 300s or lower, then I'll go on it. I don't like the idea. It's frightening to start on a medication. It's sort of an admission that I can't handle this thing on my own. I don't want to be dependent on a medication to keep me alive."

"Do you think the AZT will help you maintain a healthy lifestyle?"

"No. But it will help me maintain my T cells and help me hold off the virus."

"Okay, so you sort of envision yourself maybe gulping down the AZT with a margarita? I've got friends who do that."

"No—well, not every day. My own health-related discipline is a whole different issue. I'm not looking to AZT for help with that. That's something I have to look to myself for, at other levels than taking a pill."

"I guess I'm imagining, since I'm not on it yet either, the little ritual of taking AZT three times a day."

"See, that's my other issue with it. I have a hard time taking vitamins once a day. I had a hard time taking the naltrexone, and that was only once a day. I just don't have that kind of mentality. There are certain people who love that pill dependency, who love to be on their little pills. I went out with a guy last summer who had a little beeper. He goes everywhere with his beeper, and he's really into it."

"That used to be the rage in San Francisco. Everybody had beeper pill boxes. Was it the same in New York?"

"I guess. I'd meet people later on who would say, 'Oh God. I hear Ron's beeper all the time. Is he on AZT?' Yeah, whatever. Isn't it obvious what he has it for? What else does he have a pill beeper for?'

"I've been working with a therapist who does a lot of body manipulations. He combines spiritual, psychological, and physical work. He's very progressive and perhaps even crazy. I know that underneath it all he would never suggest that I not go on medications or anything—but he does believe that we're inundated with all kinds of viruses all the time and that if you're in a healthy state you can maintain it despite the attacks of viruses. Viruses are a constant thing in our lives anyway. We're constantly warding them off, and it looks like lots of people are doing just fine with this one. I'm not in a hurry to get on medication for any reason. It's a last-ditch effort, as far as I'm concerned. I don't mean as far as getting sick—not that last ditch. But last ditch for staying above the disease line before I start to get sick."

"So it has this symbolic—"

"Definitely it does, absolutely. Anything you have to be dependent on has a symbolic influence, and that's exactly what I'm trying to get away from, what's tugging on me. I'm trying to get to a point of independence in my life that I don't think I've ever truly reached. I'm striving for more independence and at the same time feel this pull to be dependent on a pill. I guess true independence can't really be achieved. We're all dependent on each other to some degree, but I just want to avoid that kind of dependence. I don't want to have to constantly question what the result of this or that medication is and what's the result of AIDS and what's going on. My father is on all these medications for his heart. He is trying like hell to determine—he's so out of touch anyway—but he goes through all kinds of hell trying to determine what's the side effects of the medication and what's his heart and what's gastrointestinal and what's just him feeling bad. He's in a constant state of complete anxiety."

I hadn't given much thought to parents as positive or negative role models for coping with HIV/AIDS. Except for Nathan, they seemed pretty much out of the picture for gay men I knew with asymptomatic HIV. Gay men with AIDS were certainly not the only ones suffering from the effects of "poly-pharmacy," a situation where it becomes impossible to distinguish disease symptoms from possible reactions and interactions between ten or twenty drugs, half of which the prescribing physician had usually forgotten about. As a home care nurse I often faced worried relatives who could not get their loved one to take the prescribed pile of pills four times a day. I generally pared them down to two or three and put the rest in a box.

Damian would have none of that, but his reasons were slightly different from those offered by others in this study. He didn't find promise in pharmaceuticals the way Nathan, Matthew, or Ron did, but neither were they poisons, as they were for Jason and Eric. Damian imagined that he would go on AZT someday, but he would put that day off for as long as possible. Like Kirk, Damian didn't want to be dependent on pharmaceuticals, but the issue wasn't so much being independent from pharmaceuticals as it was being more independent in general.

Unlike many of the others in this study, Damian did not anchor his decisions about HIV in any particular ideology. In fact, he didn't talk much about factors outside himself at all. He was not worried about early intervention or the quality of his positive thinking. Even as a social worker, Damian did not offer much of a cultural critique. He didn't talk about the fatalism of the press or the arrogance of the medical establishment. He did not get angry or become an AIDS activist or focus on matters such as mobilizing hope in the community.

Even Damian's holism seemed less structured, less ideological than it was for many. He didn't drink wheatgrass or worry about exercise or oxygen exchanges, but like Kirk, he avoided thinking that perfection was the answer. In so doing, Damian also avoided the guilt and blame that sometimes afflict people who decide they are totally responsible for their own health. None of the men I talked to for this study seemed to blame themselves for contracting the virus, or anyone else for that matter, and Damian was no exception. Unlike some cancer patients, they never talked about "manifesting" HIV in order to learn something important, even if they managed to do just that. No, the guilt discourse I was hearing tended to be about stress management, drug and alcohol use, not exercising or meditating enough, and perhaps current problems with adhering to safe-sex guidelines.

Damian maintained his stringent, disciplined lifestyle for only two months, although he attributed the rise in his T cells to taking better care of himself. Perhaps fear could motivate only to a point, for a while. It's certainly hard for people to keep doing the things they think they should be doing—and keep avoiding the things they shouldn't, even in the face of death. It didn't seem to me that Damian had enjoyed those two stringent, disciplined months anyway. It didn't sound as if they had been very nurturing for him.

In many ways Damian's and Kirk's stories were remarkably similar. Both paid significant attention to death. Despite holistic beliefs, both came to terms with some Western medical interventions, Kirk through taking Zovirax for herpes and Damian through undergoing a surgical procedure for something he could not spontaneously heal. In the process both confronted the limits of their thoughts and beliefs about self-healing. Neither Damian nor Kirk thought taking AZT was a good idea, but unlike Eric and Jason, they didn't think it was evil incarnate either. Both of them found ways to face facts and make adjustments without giving up their holistic beliefs.

Many of the experts in the holistic health movement have warned that strong anger or fear can actually bind us to things from which we would prefer to escape. Foucault has argued that intellectual and political activities can actually feed the forces we are trying to resist.[3] Neither Kirk nor Damian focused on factors outside of himself. Kirk used the larger social constructions and metaphors about HIV equaling contamination and death to move into himself. HIV brought "messages" about mortality, "the big D." Damian seemed to turn a reluctant and short-lived focus on the virus onto himself. In the process the metaphoric power of the virus became somewhat attenuated for both of them.

Perhaps Fire Island was attenuating some things for me as well. I had three weeks in summer 1990 to grieve memories, gather stories, and indulge a multitude of passions that refused to die. The mellow hippie who lived next door came by with some great smoke, and we took one last walk down to the western edge of the Pines where the deer—actually just the bucks—assembled every night just before sunset. The weekend crowd had shifted to the bayside for tea, but along the long strip of white sand beach I saw a few strangers scattering ashes, and I knew them.

It was time for me to go. I walked back to the harbor, past the boys at tea tapping their feet to "If you want to go to heaven, you got to raise a little hell." I walked past the mostly straight yacht crowd finishing their cocktail hour and went down the last stretch of pier. The bay rocked slowly in the sun's low embrace, exposing jades and pearl violets underneath the wavy surface. Far in the distance, another ferry headed toward Cherry Grove. Those old ferries looked so familiar—like magical friends from a 1950s storybook—and I said good-bye to them once again.

| 8 |

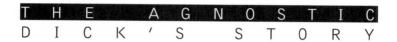

THE AGNOSTIC
DICK'S STORY

Dick was a tall, striking, Black Irish computer consultant in his midthirties. I met him at a sex club and was ecstatic that he was interested in me. We liked each other enormously, but for the most part got together only once every few months. He had a large face, the shaven parts of which seemed to shine a midnight blue as shadows played over its complex angles. Most of the time he sported one of those enormous mustaches that extend wide devilish grins down and up at the same time.

As a person Dick was unusually generous, and when I finished writing my dissertation, he reformatted it, changing the page layout, line spacing, and section headers. He taught me about styles and introduced me to small caps and the Utopia font. He also introduced me to elegant champagne—Veuve Clicquot. He was easy and natural. He did everything with style and grace but never made people feel uncomfortable. At six foot four inches and with hair that hung to the middle of his back, he was the perfect postmodern urban hippie.

Dick didn't believe that medicine had much, if anything, to offer people who were HIV positive, and he was not very interested in exploring medical alternatives either. Unlike Eric and Jason, however, he didn't rail against medicine. His skepticism never assumed ideological proportions. As will be clear in his narrative, Dick's reluctance to embrace Western medicine was not a result of fear or denial. Nor was it because he shared Eric's sociological understanding of power and medicine or Jason's mind-over-matter approach to health. Even though I sense that Dick would have shared many of Eric's and Jason's other views, these were not at all central to his story.

Dick was in many ways like my best friend, Gabe. Both were deeply rooted in their own lives, their own self-understandings, and their own practices. Both were well educated, well informed, and well integrated into their communities. Both were also delightful storytellers, and I looked forward to our talk, which took place in my living room.

▼ ▼ ▼

"It's been a while since the last time I talked to you. I'm trying to remember what the idea is."

"The idea is that I'd like for you to tell me, in twenty-five words or less, how HIV has affected your life. You can start anywhere you want and talk about anything that you want. Eventually the whole story will come together, whether chronologically or in any other way."

"Boy, what a big subject! Well, HIV really affected my life directly when I had my antibody test, which I did when the person that I loved the most in the world was in New Zealand, a long way away, dying from AIDS. I decided it was finally time to face certain facts and get tested myself. I was very concerned with the issues of insurability and employability. Those were the two things I thought would be most affected by a positive outcome. The idea that I'd probably never be able to get health insurance and would probably also never be hired by anyone again did not appeal to me!" he laughed. "So I arranged all these layers of anonymity around what I was doing. I actually went to New York and got my friend who was a doctor to draw my blood and have it tested anonymously by the city health department. It just so happened that the department of the hospital that he ran provided the AIDS assessment service. So I thought, yes, I'll go three thousand miles away, and I'll do it anonymously, and it will be done by friends, and that way whatever comes out, only I will know.

"So I went to great lengths to preserve secrecy, which sounds a bit silly today, but actually in 1987 it wasn't quite so silly. William Buckley was saying things about tattooing people with the AIDS virus, and there were a whole lot of issues about employability and insurability. It was very important to feel safe about privacy issues because there were some very real dangers with identifying oneself or, more importantly, allowing oneself to be identified as an 'AIDS carrier.' So those were the things that I was thinking about when I decided to be tested. And my dear friend Dr. Paul, who is now deceased from AIDS, asked me how I wanted it. I told him, 'Just take the results, put them in an envelope, address them to me without comment, and mail them to my home in San Francisco.' I think his ethical nature wanted to make sure that I had some kind of posttesting counseling. It was very nice of him not to superimpose his opinion about how I should be treated over my opinion about how I wanted to be treated. Our friendship was such that he agreed to do it my way.

"What I didn't know was that Paul was also antibody positive at the time. I remember the day the envelope came. He wrote on the bottom of the test report: 'I know how you feel. Call me if you want.' That 'I know how you feel' meant 'I'm in this boat, too; you're not the only person who is going through this.' He was a wonderful, empathetic person. He said very little, but it was exactly the right thing and it conveyed a great deal."

"So did you call him?"

"Not right away. I thought about it for a while. I was not surprised about the result. I figured that a positive outcome was a foregone conclusion, and that's why I had not bothered to test for so long—not because I was in any sort of denial but quite the reverse. I was thinking, I've got to be infected because so many of my lovers are dead and so are many people who did the very same things I did. It only made sense that I would have been infected in the course of my behaviors. So it was not a shock. I wasn't thinking, oh, this couldn't be happening. I was thinking, of course, this is happening, you fool; what did you think was going to happen?"

He started laughing and replied, "So I thought about it for a while and went through what was probably a fairly standard series of reactions in rapid succession. You feel like—oh no, this must be a mistake; then, well, no, maybe it really is true; then making deals with God like, please let this not be true and I'll never have sex again as long as I live. I had about one to five minutes with each of these reactions in the course of the first day of knowing. I ran through that whole gamut of things pretty quickly and experienced each one deeply but briefly. Finally I thought, oh, this is ridiculous. It was funny—I think I probably felt all of the things that anybody's ever felt who gets a positive test result, especially in 1987, when it was translated as, you're dead; you're a ticking bomb just walking around waiting to go off. And then you're going to die horribly, and probably slowly!"

"Where did you hear that HIV was a ticking time bomb?"

"I decided that the progression was: antibody positive, diagnosis, death. An awful lot of people I knew had recently gone through those three stages. The thing that affected me most at the time, probably more than anything that's ever happened in my life, was the death of Peter. He was from New Zealand, and I met him here in the U.S. through a mutual friend. We became the very, very best of friends. He was the human being with whom I had the closest relationship in my life. It was way more than lovers. It was just this incredible connection in so many ways. I think we sort of had sex once, but it was just kind of peripheral to something else that was going on. We were extremely close. We saw each other every day. We knew everything about each other's lives. He had boyfriends and I had boyfriends, and we knew all about and talked to each other about our boyfriends—so we were more intimate with each other than we were with our respective lovers. It would take me more tape than is available and more time than I have to try to describe the wonderfulness of that relationship. Experiencing how wonderful and pure a love between two men can be stands as the high-water mark in my life. I am very fortunate to have had that experience in life with a man. I think if you get one of those, you're doing real good. If people have that once, they are very lucky. If it happens more than once, you're exceptional."

"For me that happened once, with Gabe."

"Things like that are rare. I cared more about Peter than anyone I had ever known before or since. The pattern that things took in 1987 became defined for me through Peter's experience. He was going through the progression: antibody positive, diagnosis, death. He was close to death then. AZT was still—nobody was quite sure what that was all about. I seem to remember people doing egg lecithin and AL-721 and drugs that you don't hear about anymore because they didn't work. A lot of people were trying a lot of things, and nobody was getting better. People were only dying. So that's why I decided that that was the inevitable course of events after getting a positive antibody test—that one would sooner or later get sick and then die quite prematurely, and not in a particularly attractive manner. And that was how I determined what that particular piece of news meant for me.

"I didn't really freak out or go crazy; I just got coldly practical about it because that's usually how I react to emergencies. I could either spend a lot of time wailing and gnashing my teeth, or I could make certain decisions about how I would live my life. A lot of my decision making had to do with how I would live, where I would live, who I would live with, what kind of work I would do, what the nature of the structure of my life would be, where I would go, how much time I would spend there, what priorities I'd have. I thought a lot about my priorities and basically came up with issues that I had always been working on anyway.

"I was never particularly success or career oriented. I tried to have the way I made money be a vehicle for my enjoyment of life. For me that usually means travel and having lots of leisure time to pursue things that interest me—time to read books that I think are interesting rather than books on subjects that I need to know for my work—stuff like that. I wanted to go on train rides that lasted for days and just sit and read in a moving train car.

"I couldn't picture myself applying for a 'permanent job' and going through any kind of health screening for group life insurance because I figured that would turn up the fact of my antibody status. I decided to continue with my freelance business and not try to get a job since I was potentially unemployable and uninsurable anyway. All this sounds weird to me as I sit here and say it; it sounds like the ravings of a paranoid—but just a very short couple of years ago all of those things were very real considerations. People were being fired from jobs or dropped by their insurance carriers. One week's headline was about some queen whose insurance company dropped her like a hot potato the first time she sent in a claim for some AIDS-related treatment. People were being fired from their jobs instantly on the very rumor that they had AIDS—for example, people in food handling. That was one of the issues at the time—whether all food-handling people should be tested for antibodies and, if positive, immediately fired to protect the public health.

"I read these things in the only sources of information about AIDS at the time, the gay media. The straight media was still not doing anything terribly in depth in those days. In 1987 they were more concerned with what Vanna White was wearing on television. More print was going to subjects like that than to how gay men were dealing with AIDS-related discrimination. That was the Zeitgeist, the AIDS Zeitgeist that I emerged into as an antibody-positive person. It was a scary place. There wasn't much that was hopeful about it. It was a pretty grim picture. I basically got my induction notice to join the ranks of those who had gone before me to get sick and die. It was like, okay, now you're in it, too. Now AIDS is no longer a theoretical issue. Now it has just hit your personal life in a very close-up and personal way.

"How all that unfolded over the past two and a half years was that I continued to be alive and well and healthy. I reaffirm the fact that life is a miracle and every minute of it is very much worth loving. The clouds have sort of lifted from my whole being over the last two and a half years, but it was a very slow and gradual process, sort of like a San Francisco day, when it's really foggy in the morning and it gets almost imperceptibly lighter, so that by lunchtime it's finally sunny. An awful lot of people—I never dreamed I could love people that much—have been jerked or ripped or torn out of my life, which has left scars that will never heal. But instead of letting those experiences all be reasons to be angry and bitter and old before my time, I managed to translate them into reasons to be happy, into feeling lucky to be alive and appreciating just how much of a miracle life is, on a daily basis for the rest of my life, however long that lasts.

"So I started out being really scared. I had a very gloomy outlook on life in general in that it was all darkened by the fact that I was walking around as a quote unquote carrier. It's so much like *The Scarlet Letter*, carrying the Big 'A'; you're infected. I hated that, but I'm still alive. I'm still well. I'm in a community of people who are all in the same boat as me. I'm in the best place in the world that I could be. I've lived lots of other places since I've been infected. I've been in New York and back here in San Francisco and a lot of different places. My gay brothers that I see in other places are not doing as well or being as well served as the people right here at home. So I think that it could be a whole lot worse."

"How long did you feel like you were wearing the Scarlet Letter?"

"It was a long time, at least the first year."

"Where did you feel that? Did you feel that in the gay community?"

"It was not diminished even amongst other gay people. Ever since I was in high school, I've read the personal ads in papers like the Village Voice because I was always endlessly fascinated by what people are looking for. I read the want ads every Sunday, too, whether I'm looking for work or not, just because I want to stay in touch with what people are looking for. Then antibody status became one of the necessary statistics that one included in a capsule description of oneself in a personal ad. It used to be eyes, hair, built or not built, cut or uncut, active/passive—all these things. Then at some point antibody status started to appear as a criterion, as an immediate measurable indicator of one's desirability to others of one's kind. So that reinforced the feeling—now you're in the out-group; now you're in the 'B' group, honey; all these ads that say, 'Antibody-positives need not apply.'

"As a white man in America I had never been in a group that need not apply for anything. I don't think I ever thought of myself as a second-class citizen because of being gay because that was largely overridden by the fact that as a white male in American society I was born to the privileged class. The world was set up for me. I was in the 'A' group just by my birthright—white, speak English, big dick, young. It was perfect. People sit around over coffee and invent people like I thought I was in terms of those kinds of criteria. So suddenly I encountered my first experience ever of not being in the 'A' group anymore."

"Did you feel it anywhere else other than the want ads? You don't strike me as the type who would really look for relationships in the want ads."

"No. Because the person that I loved the most was dying, I was convinced that love itself was dying and that I would never care about or have relationships of any significance again. I would probably just get sick and die anyway. That was probably how things were going to go.

"And then Peter died, and I went to New Zealand. We had a pact. When he knew he was going to die, he would tell me, and I would come and see him again before he did. We were separated because he had to go back to his own country when he got sick. As an illegal alien he couldn't get treated or feel safe about having a fatal disease here. He had to go home. We corresponded as his disease progressed, and I have a wonderful collection of letters about what we thought was happening to us at the time. In fact, I just came upon them the day before yesterday and read them all again on the occasion of another friend's death. I thought, oh my God, here are Peter's letters. What a perfect day to find them. I'll just read them again because I think I can handle it now. And it was great. I didn't cry at all. I just felt very nice.

"That was what was going on at the time. I thought that love itself was dying along with him. And he did die, but as much as I thought that I never would, I did get over it. I did get over it. For a whole year black was my primary wardrobe color, and I generally dress quite colorfully, but black was also the general color of my mood. I was pretty serious about an awful lot of things. At that time I was driving an hour each way to work, and I would play sad music on the tape deck in the car and cry by myself as I drove back and forth. That's how I spent my commuting time, in personal grief work, because I don't manage that stuff very well publicly. I think grief is an intensely personal thing, and I frustrate people who think it's their job to comfort me when I'm grieving because I truly do want to be left alone. I have to do that myself. And I will. Then I'll get over it and be fine, but it takes a while.

"So it was perfect. I had two hours a day locked in this tin can rolling down the freeway to work on—I don't know what. I don't think my goal was to be happy again because I still thought that I would never be happy again. I think that my goal was just to achieve some kind of peace, and I separated that from being happy. I think that one can be at peace or calm and still carry the permanent leaded weight of deep grief. But I don't think that one can be happy quite in the innocent way that I had felt myself to be happy before. Peter's death was where I lost my last shred of innocence.

"As you get older, I think that the experiences of life can chip away at one's sense of wonder or good nature or one's feeling that the world is a safe and happy place in which everything nice is going to happen to you and you are going to be fulfilled and everything's going to be good. I started out thinking that, but the feeling deteriorates over time. When Peter died, the last scrap of belief in the world as a safe and happy place disintegrated. I just didn't believe that anymore."

"Is there a safe and happy place beyond the world for you?"

"No. I don't have any comforting set of spiritual notions. I was raised as a dogmatic Catholic by not particularly well-educated Irish and Scottish first-generation American parents who didn't go to college and didn't think critically. All of my primary and high school education was by nuns, so it was a sort of Baltimore Catechism kind of childhood. I didn't buy their thinking—when you are young and stupid, you think life is pretty; then you grow up and find out that it isn't; then you die, and the sweet by and by is where everything will be cool again. I could never swallow all that. Along about the time I achieved the age of reason, I figured out that religion was a system that had been invented by humans to give them power over other humans. This whole bit about reward and punishment and saving up grace as though it were a bank account that could be cashed in for favors at the end of your life struck me as too much like a monetary system to have any kind of spiritual significance. So I jettisoned a lot of that luggage without feeling the necessity to replace it with some other spiritual system. Catholics think that you're here to suffer and you get paid off when it's over. I think that I'm here to have a good time, and I'm not going to take my chances that there might be an afterlife where things will be better. I want things to be good here.

"I am basically a fairly positive person who likes himself and likes his life and is fairly self-confident and enjoys having a good time. Somebody charted my planets for me once, and I have seven out of nine planets in Leo, you know, Leo with a Leo rising. So I'm out for a good time. You know what all that is. I couldn't stay miserable forever. Yet the first year after Peter died was the longest year of my whole life. I was miserable all the time, and life was just black. Then over the period of the second year it got grayer, progressively lighter, and in the last half year or so I think that I got a hell of a lot happier than I was then. Not like I was before it happened because that was a sort of childish innocence based on ignorance. I don't feel that sort of youthful notion that everything's going to get better as I go along, that I'm in the prime of my life, I'm going to conquer the world. Now I realize that death happens and things end, but I think that one can know that and be happy anyway.

"To draw on an old Catholic metaphor, it's sort of like the fall from grace. Before they got knowledge, Adam and Eve had this sort of blissful ignorance where everything was always perfect and they didn't know anything other. But then they got knowledge, which changed everything and got them thrown out of the good situation they were in. That's sort of what happened to me. Now I know what death is. I have the knowledge of death, so I feel older and wiser. I'm certain that I will never have the innocent quality of happiness I had before I knew of death, but I think it is still possible for me to be happy anyway.

"I'm not sure how or why I came to that conclusion. This is probably the first time I've ever articulated what I think about a lot of these things. A lot of it has been bouncing around in my head for a while, but I never actually put it together, codified it into a view of life, or presented it to anyone. So I don't know if any of this will make sense when it's played back, but I feel like I'm making sense to myself now as I say it."

Dick's concise account of regaining a kind of happiness after losing the love of his life makes enormous sense. Dick's relationship with Peter suggests Kierkegaard's idea of world-defining commitments, which

Kierkegaard thought were vitally necessary to any rich and full life.[1] Although Dick's loss shared some elements with Matthew's loss of his lover, Dick cannot even imagine a new relationship, a replacement. For Dick, love is not an abstract concept or a force that somehow attaches itself to a beloved object. Love is a particular embodied experience, so when Peter died, love died as well.

To avoid commitments like Dick's love of Peter is to avoid life itself. But world-defining commitments come with a price. They must eventually be mourned. That is the essential process with which Dick was coming to terms. Thus trying to distinguish between the happiness he felt before and after coming to know death was not simply an abstract philosophical issue for Dick. It was about distinguishing who he was as a man who had lived, loved, and mourned. Dick was not alone in this struggle. Freud, Kierkegaard, Becker, and Wilbur all worked on making sense out of mourning and mortality without recourse to overly simple religious or New Age explanations.[2]

▼ ▼ ▼

"So here I am. I'm thirty-four and still alive, and there are some decisions before me about what to do. I went through this whole bit about whether to take the test or not. I finally made a decision, got tested, and spent a long time coping with the aftermath of that decision. Now that that's over, it's time for me to decide if I want to start monitoring T cells. And based on that information, do I want to start doing prophylaxis of some sort? Do I want to start employing aggressive techniques to try to stave off the onset of AIDS?

"I hear a lot of hopeful things. I spoke to somebody last week who told me that in a month there will be some results published about compound Q and peptide T which are very hopeful. We have all heard rumors of therapies that have been at one point or another very hopeful for quite a few years now, but we're all still dying! So that's where that gets you. Hope lets you continue to live, but it's hope tempered by the fact that nothing has proven to pan out in terms of an effective therapy or a cure. So I'm sort of guardedly hopeful or cynically hopeful."

"We're not all dying."

"I know that we're not all dying. But everyone I love is dying or dead. This is personal. I'm not being scientific. My world is destroyed. It will never be the same again. For better or worse, Peter's death changed me profoundly. So I'm very glad that we're not all dying, that I'm not dying. And that's why I'm happier than I was a couple of years ago. Nevertheless, my past is disappearing before my eyes. All of my pals who knew me and were part of my experience in San Francisco aren't around anymore. There's no witness to my life."

"I know what you mean by that. There are only a few left for me—and most of them are HIV positive."

"Yep. We're living on borrowed time or walking around ticking or whatever. Realizing that has had a lot to do with my getting happy again. I have had a very inordinate amount of death amongst the men that I love—father, best friend, all my lovers, who have also been men. The women don't seem to die, but men die on me, starting with my dad when I was nineteen and continuing for so long. My dad went through what people with AIDS go through. He was forty-nine. In the last year of his life his aging accelerated so that when he died, he looked like a very old man, both because of the cancer and the things they tried to fix it with. He lost a lot of weight, his hair fell out, he went into the hospital and came out and went into the hospital—and then never came out again.

"I didn't know then that that was going to be a rehearsal for a huge part of the rest of my life. I thought it was an isolated incident. Then my best friend committed suicide a couple of years after that. So when AIDS started happening to me in my early thirties, I'd already had some experience with close loved ones dying from long, debilitating diseases. That's just what happened to me, and it doesn't mean anything beyond myself. If one person would get better, I might be more hopeful. That's all it would take. But I haven't seen that happen."

"What do you mean by 'get better'?"

"If I would just see somebody get sick and get well and stay well, instead of starting a cycle and getting sick and then getting sick again and then getting sick more and more frequently and then getting sick and just staying that way."

▼ ▼ ▼

I have often asked people what they meant by "getting better" or "surviving HIV or AIDS" or "beating it." What I generally discover is that people often use the language without giving much thought to what they mean. The unconscious or unfocused thought behind the phrases is usually broader and grander than what they finally end up telling me. When "beating AIDS" means T cells increasing to 1200 or the antibody test somehow changing to negative, almost no one beats it. Nobody survives. But when surviving means living longer than the projected "average" time from infection to AIDS or surviving the first and second waves of AIDS deaths in one's own community or finally making that trip to Bali, then survival is widespread.

Dick did not see survival in his community. All of his men were dying or dead. Dick's definition of survival didn't really include asymptomatics like himself. Indeed, his community's definition of survival used to be like Dick's. The poster boy "survivors" were those who had AIDS for five years or more, but none of them ever "got better and stayed well." They just rebounded from their several bouts with illness. The length of time HIV-positive people stayed healthy was not how survival was defined, not by the industry and not by people like Dick. Matthew's long-term survival with HIV (in 1998, twenty years) did not provide an instance of "survival" for many. So Dick interpreted his own situation with asymptomatic HIV infection as one that would eventually look like the experiences of his friends: HIV positive to AIDS to death. I asked him what he thought about HIV-positive people who weren't getting sick, such as himself.

▼ ▼ ▼

"Yeah, what about that? I think that I die a little bit every day. It will just be a long time before it manifests itself as something identifiable. I try to be really honest with myself. I don't think I feel physically worse than I did when I was young and healthy—or thought I was healthy, because I don't know how long I've been infected. It could have been as long as ten or thirteen years ago, between 1977 and 1980. I came out in New York in 1977—you know, the balcony of the Saint, the St. Mark's Baths, and the bushes of Fire Island. That was 1977 to 1980. Then I moved to San Francisco and was at Eighth and Howard and Rich Street on a daily basis for years.[3]

"So it happened at least seven years ago, and if the things I read are true, things will start to happen in about ten years. So I don't think, yeah, I'm HIV positive, but I'm staying well. I think, well, it's six years out, it's seven years out, and I'm a little less well than I was the year before, but the cumulative effect won't be apparent for a while yet.

That's how I'm feeling. I pay real close attention to myself. I'm always looking for the little potential KS lesion or the first sign of mold in the back of my throat." He laughed. "Not mold, fungus."

"Thrush?"

"Thrush? What's thrush?"

"Yeast."

"Right. It's not mold or fungus; it's yeast! You know what I mean. I look for all those things. I watch my coloring and how fast my hair is falling out. And, of course, at my age some of those things start to happen anyway, so I don't know how much of that to attribute to aging or whether it's just the little signs."

"The big 'A' or the little 'a'?"

"That's good. Yeah, the big 'A' or the little 'a'? I haven't heard that before. That's good. So on days when I'm being rational and sane, I think, oh, shut up, no big deal. Other days I think, this is just a little indicator that I'm getting sicker. So to get past that, the thing to do is to get some facts. The big issue for me now is to count T cells or not to count T cells.

"If I start counting T cells, I'd probably put numbers on a spreadsheet that I could graph and make a line chart. On days when the line went up, I might look at it and think, I'll feel good today. On days when it went down, I'll feel like I'm going down. My bottom line is this: I am trying to postpone—or altogether avoid—organizing my feelings about myself and the world around having AIDS. I don't want to take AZT with that damn pillbox with the buzzer, so that every four hours out of every twenty-four-hour day the buzzer will go off and jerk me out of whatever I'm doing. I don't want to be continually reminded that I'm sick or have to take medicine or have to get my T cells counted and plotted. I don't want to freak out when they start to go down, then feel sick, then get sick and begin the whole downward spiral.

"I really think that intangible things like visualization count for as much as things like taking AZT. If I start to link the way I feel about myself to some number on a bar chart, then that will start to rule my life. When the numbers go down, my ability to feel well and good will go down. I might get up feeling great on a nice sunny day and get out my computer and check my latest numbers and notice that they've been declining over a while. Then my day will be ruined. I just don't want to build a great deal of my personal Zeitgeist around that data."

▼ ▼ ▼

Like many of the others I interviewed, Dick thought "intangible things like visualization" counted. Dick did not want to graph his health on a spreadsheet. The numbers simply did not fit into his calculations. He was afraid that the picture itself might be as detrimental to his health as the virus. Although he tried to discount these data bits, they had such powerful meanings for Dick that he was afraid they might obliterate the way he felt about himself and his world. If Dick linked his T-cell counts with how he felt, the T-cell counts might have overcome his self-understanding and come to "rule" his life. Eric, Jason, and Damian all had similar fears.

One powerful and pervasive symbol of our newly medicalized lives was the battery-powered beeping pillbox. Initially, patients were supposed to take their AZT every four hours around the clock. The disease was so horrible and so frightening that few people questioned the wisdom of waking up in the middle of the night to take a pill—even though its efficacy and optimal dosage had never been established. As a nurse I advised people from the beginning to skip the night dose or to take three pills before bed and three in the morning. The twelve-pills-a-day regime, divided rigorously into six equal intervals, came out of somebody's head, not from research studies, and many people carried around beeper boxes to make sure they did it right. This is exactly the sort of thing that many in our community were defending themselves against.

▼ ▼ ▼

"Now you've got to help me a bit," I continued. "This is the part I'm most perplexed by. I've noticed that people who don't want to do their T cells, and then finally do them anyway, often fulfill their prophecies about them. They wind up paying more attention to the numbers than those who aren't so reluctant. I'm wondering if you don't know something about yourself or the way you would respond to those numbers."

"I don't know. I think fear is a very reasonable assumption here. If I've been gradually dropping T cells over the last few years, I don't really want to be reminded of that fact or have it verified. I knew I was antibody positive when I got the test, and after taking it, I was bummed out for a long time. I suspect that my T cells may be declining. Maybe they are; maybe they aren't. What I ask myself is, what practical good will it do me to know? What benefit is to be gained? What unpleasantness is to occur? Profit/loss. Let's look at this the way I look at everything else."

"Okay—tell me what the balance sheet shows."

"And the balance sheet says there's not a great deal to be gained because if your T cells are going down, there isn't a fucking thing you can do about it. It's not like it would confirm or deny that I have some disease that there's something you can do for it. There isn't. I could take a highly toxic drug called AZT that will eat my bone marrow and build for me the 'ill person' Zeitgeist by putting me on this permanent prescription that I'll never get off of, which would also identify me as an HIVer to the insurance companies to whom I have to send the AZT bills, which would get me put on the list of people who should be executed or sent to concentration camps or whatever. So all of that is to be lost. And identifying myself as a sick person—both publicly and to myself—would seriously hurt my sense of well-being. I stand to lose that if I get into searching for confirmation that I have some preliminary manifestation of AIDS.

"Even so, from the minute you get diagnosed as HIV positive to the minute you die, it's all having AIDS, as far as I'm concerned. It's just a question of degree. You've got AIDS. It's just a continuum, and you're on it from the minute you get diagnosed. So part of me laughs at myself and says, honey, you are in heavy denial; you're trying to preserve this fragile illusion that you're really not sick or that you really don't have AIDS, an illusion that's getting progressively more fragile. And maybe I am, but that's what it takes for me to get up every day and keep living. If I start counting T cells, that will probably lead me to start taking medicine. If I start counting T cells and taking medicine, I'm going to become like some hypochondriac old lady who gets worried and obsessed and then wants to talk about it all the time. It's boring!

"I want to spend my energy making sure that the quality of my life, however much longer it's going to be, is as high as I can possibly make it. I do work that I really enjoy. I love being a teacher because I feel like I can start people out doing something that will continue after I'm gone. I may have somebody for only one day, but I may be able to plant some kind of seed or light some kind of spark in them that will make their life better. I think that's kind of neat. I feel like I'm giving a little something back to somebody somewhere for all the good things I have taken from living. I've had a wonderful, marvelous, incredibly lucky life. I've met wonderful people and have had things happen to me that I had no reason to think I deserved. So I want to do those sorts of things instead of sitting around fussing over whether my T cells went up or down."

"Do you know anybody who is monitoring T cells, taking AZT, and not being a hypochondriac?"

"No. One of my friends has been watching his T cells decline for a long time. As a result, he started taking AZT. We were sitting around, and he was describing how much weirder and worse he feels now that he's started taking a strange and powerful new drug. So, yeah, watch your T cells decline, take AZT, feel weird, get the idea planted in your head that you're sick, pay too much attention to yourself. It just gets in your way. It gets in the way of doing whatever else you try to do in your day."

"Okay. Have you been presented with the evangelical medical appeal?"

"My friend the doctor tried to give me that. I just buried him last month in New York. So, heal thyself, physician. Yeah, I've had people do that and turn around and die themselves. Chinese herbalists—dead. Western medicine—dead. Clean living, bodybuilding, good diet, lots of exercise—dead. Every damn one of them. So anybody can get evangelical in my face about anything they want, and I'll listen to them and go, 'Yeah, okay, fine. Show me a live one and we'll talk.'"

"I still have the feeling that what you're hearing, what the community is hearing, may be bleaker than it is."

"Well, bleaker than it might be. It also could just be my personal reaction. How I feel or how I decide what to do is not just based on hard information or facts. It's based on a lot of intangible stuff."

Dick seemed to reject both biomedicine and the narrative accounts of survival in our community, and his approach seemed needlessly myopic and even deadly. It flew in the face of my rationalism and my idealism. Perhaps Dick needed to hear Matthew's story, but for every Matthew there was at least one Peter, and Peter was the one he loved.

Although Dick had little hope in medicine or New Age holism, he could not wholly abandon hope because he knew that he needed hope to keep living. His hope was tempered by his experience, which was that HIV invariably led to AIDS and AIDS invariably led to death. I was concerned that his personal experience with HIV was nonetheless essentially hopeless, at least as far as either alternative interventions or Western medicine was concerned. But Dick's hopes were not about medicine or prolonging biological life. Dick's hope was about preserving what was valuable to him in his own life.

▼▼▼

"Besides all that, tell me what's happened with sex."

"I used to enjoy sex tremendously. I was built for sex. I was born for sex. I think most of the people I've had sex with would agree." He laughed. "I have not enjoyed sex the way I used to since I found out that I was antibody positive because I had this incredible experience. I was actually right in the middle of fucking someone way back in the beginning of this, around 1983, and I actually saw death as I was fucking this person. It was like an equation, SEX = DEATH, and it occurred to me in an almost visual way. I still remember it very clearly to this day. Things have not been the same since, but it was confirmed and made permanent when I got my antibody test.

"I have a great deal of control, and I am now afraid to lose control. Sex used to be the place where you could rip the lid off, pull your brains out, throw them against the wall, watch it splash, and feel that incredible feeling that only comes when you really give it all up. I have not allowed myself to feel that since I knew that I was infected because now even safe sex is something that could kill someone."

"So what's safe sex about for you?"

"Safe sex is the best we can get. It's a substitute for just plain sex. Safe sex is a pale imitation of what sex used to be. The thing about sex, before it became safe sex, was abandon. Safe sex is sex without abandon.

"It doesn't have a great deal to do with a list of acts that one does or does not perform. It has to do with the attitude or approach one takes to doing them. I still do the same things I ever did, largely, but I have an almost out-of-body experience when I'm having sex, where I feel like I'm above myself watching myself have sex. One portion of my consciousness is always separated and overseeing what's going on. That's what I mean about sex without abandon. It is not possible for me to lose myself—to become subsumed in a moment of sexual communion— because there is one part of me that always has to be the superego and stay in charge and not go off because that might mean that I do something life threatening. The supervisor always has to be on duty.

"It's not a big deal. It's not like sex is ruined for me or that I don't enjoy it anymore or I do it any less. It's all fine. It's just changed. Like I said, I've changed irrevocably for better or worse, and one of the things that's changed is my awareness of things, including myself. Now I can be doing something and watch myself doing it at the same time and experience both of those states of consciousness simultaneously. Before it was possible for me to become subsumed or even consumed in the flame of passion. I haven't experienced that in a long time. I like to think that it's possible, but I am sure that it's not likely."

"I want to know about the supervisor. What does he permit? What does he forbid? What does he give you a hard time about?"

"I am not into condoms. I don't enjoy using condoms. They greatly reduce the amount of pleasure I get from sex. Unfortunately, my favorite thing to do is fuck. In 1990 you just can't do that without condoms, or if you do, and sometimes I do, I have to make sure that I don't ejaculate. So one of the supervisor's jobs is to make sure that no matter how much fun you're having or how excruciatingly close to orgasm you are, it must be physically impossible to ejaculate while you're inside somebody else. It's almost a conditioned response that requires me to pull out when I know that I'm going to cum. I am pleased to say that in several years of having lots of sex with and without rubbers, but a lot of it without, that I've never lost control and cum in somebody and thought, oh my God, now I've killed this person.

"So the supervisor's main function is to make sure that I don't get so selfishly carried away with my own physical gratification that I place any other person at any kind of health risk. That's his job—to make sure that I don't do anything stupid like place my paltry gratification over the value of another person's life."

"If you're still fucking without condoms, do you still or did you ever make routine visits to the City Clinic?"

"I had STDs [sexually transmitted diseases] twice. I had genital gonorrhea, a dripping dick, for like a day, and I knew immediately what it was. The minute it started dripping, I went to the clinic and got some antibiotics and cured myself. That was it. That happened on two occasions a year apart in 1981 and 1982. And that was that. Now I hardly even think about STDs anymore because I hope that coitus interruptus is something that reduces the possibility of that sort of thing."

"I don't think so."

"But I have a lot less partners, and everybody's so health conscious now. I think we're all paying a lot more attention to that sort of thing.

Whereas if I was going to take a half a Quaalude and a few lines of blow and go down to Eighth and Howard and literally fuck ten or fifteen people before I got home, I should think my chances of picking up an STD would be much higher in an environment like that.

"One of the few things I've gained from all this is the joy of selectivity. When I do fuck now, it's usually somebody I really want to, whereas before I would just do it at the drop of a hat because it was there. I think if I practiced more, condoms would be easier, but instead I generally have sex with just a couple of people, and we mutually agree that we are not going to use them and that I'm just not going to cum in them and that's it."

▼▼▼

Obviously, Dick did not easily submit to the prescriptive norms of the health establishment. He was not any more interested in condoms than he had been in counseling after his HIV test. It wasn't that he was unaware or unable to make changes. Whereas some in the community went on sexually as if nothing had changed, Dick was not one of these. Sex did change for Dick. In fact, it changed more for Dick than it did for many of those who accepted each public health recommendation intellectually but could not consistently follow through in their lives.

Dick's decision to continue having sex without condoms (but with far fewer partners who were no longer anonymous) and without ejaculation had its own internal reasoning. Although forgoing condoms increased his risk for some STDs, his risk for intestinal parasites decreased far more than if he had continued to be very promiscuous with condoms. Whereas his HIV-positive partners were at increased risk for additional exposure to HIV, Dick's behavior produced less of that particular risk than, for instance, using condoms 90 percent of the time with partners who ejaculated inside or even 100 percent of the time with condoms that occasionally break.[4]

▼▼▼

"This has been real helpful for me," Dick continued. "Peter died seven thousand miles away, and I never really got to talk a lot about what happened to me when he died. I have lost a lot of significant people. What do you do? Talk to their bereaved lover about how much you miss them? It's really hard to do that. Peter was the most beautiful person that many people had ever seen physically. He was just perfect, and he worked in a gym, so there was all that, too. A whole lot of people in town had a whole lot of trips about Peter that had much more to do with their own feelings than they had to do with him. So when I knew that he was dying in New Zealand, I absented myself from San Francisco and lived in New York for six months because I didn't want these fools to stagger up to me on the street and act out their drama about how they felt about him dying in my face. I thought, the first person that does that, I'm going to deck 'em. I'm going to rip their face off. I had to go away from all that.

"When he finally did die, I grieved privately as I am wont to do, but I have always missed the opportunity to talk about it a little bit. I was alone when he died, and I stayed alone for months afterward, and by the time I got back here, it had all sort of died down. That was for the better because I knew it was going to be really hard to deal with my own feelings. I knew that if I were here, a lot of people would want me to help them deal with their feelings, and I knew that I didn't have the resources to do that."

"You never went to a widows' group or a support group?"

"It wasn't official. We were never married."

"I never went either. I just couldn't see it."

"I did start writing to my mother, who likes to think that she has a close family, but we're Irish and we don't talk about things that upset anyone. We keep everything on the surface. I wrote to her that my best friend had just died horribly and I didn't feel very good. All I wanted her to say was, 'I'm sorry your friend died.' Instead she said stupid things like 'Oh, that's how you might die. Maybe you want to rethink your existence. Isn't it a pity that people make bad choices and have to deal with the consequences.' And I was like, wait a minute! All you had to say was, 'I'm really sorry that somebody you loved died. You must feel bad.' That's all I wanted."

"She knows you're gay?"

"I haven't told her, but if she doesn't know, it's part of that process of making everything nice all the time. It's because she refuses to know. I think she knew I was queer before I was five years old and got kind of scared about that. She's Catholic, and most of her self-definition comes from being a Catholic mother, which is a very rigid set of criteria, one of which is you don't produce queer children because that is a failure of sorts. Consequently, she can't acknowledge that she has queer children because that would mean that she failed at the one thing that gives her all her self-value.

"I'm not mad at her because she's only being who she is. She's a sixty-year-old lady. She's not going to change the way she thinks now, but I felt so alone. I made a decision not to spend the rest of my life writing letters to my mother telling her what the weather was like or what I had for breakfast. If she asks, 'How are you?' then I'm going to tell her. I tell her when somebody I love dies or that I spent all last week going to visit a friend in the hospital before work, so I'm kind of tired. I tell her because she asks, and the stuff she gives me back just really disappoints me. I always thought she was pretty smart, but now I'm not so sure.

"But the price I paid for dealing with Peter's death in the way that I did was not having anyone who ever even knew who he was, who he was to me. I just got up every day and went to work and was distracted. I didn't talk a whole lot. People would ask, 'What's the matter with you?' and I'd want to say, 'What the fuck do you think is the matter with me? All the light in my whole world just went out forever, and that's what's the matter with me. Thanks for asking!'

"So this has been very nice for me. Thank you for the opportunity to talk about it. I've been carrying that around with me for a long time. You're lucky. You have people you can talk to."

"Two or three. It's weird; a lot of people never knew Steve or Duckus. There are such rapid changes here. People are new to the gym, or they didn't know them because they've only been in San Francisco three or four years."

"Yeah. Two years is a lifetime in San Francisco. Peter's been dead for two years. He's been gone for three. It might as well be a hundred. I used to know all his boyfriends, but I don't see those guys anymore. I know for certain that some of them are dead, too."

"I met Steve when I was twenty-five and was with him until I was thirty. I see his brother and a college friend of his in New York sometimes. I call his mother every now and then, and that's my connection to Steve, a man that I spent almost six years with and then three after that. Almost nobody knows. Nobody knows him."

"That's so weird. It's like me feeling that my past is vanishing. It's like it didn't happen. Nobody even knows. I mean how could you have such an incredibly significant part of your life—nine years with Steve—and now not have anything to reflect that it ever existed?"

"Me."

"That's it. When all that's left is yourself, it's really strange.

| 9 |

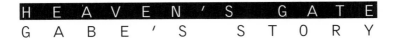

GABE'S STORY

The West used to measure its history in monarchical reigns. When the merchant class became the predominant force in the world, Western time was converted into decades and centuries. Yet the new intervals continued to be defined by human events. Often the centuries and decades adhered to the rulers and became no more regular or predictable than the length of a new monarch's reign. The nineteenth century waited for Victoria and then died with her. Eisenhower ushered in the security of the 1950s, which ended with the Kennedy assassination and Vietnam. But taken as a whole, Western history stretches itself out like those time lines that decorate grade-school classrooms. Even our mystical time runs like a great highway from the Creation to the Passion to the Last Judgment.

The Chinese perceive their time in smaller measures, rigorously regular and as predictable as the sun's progression toward the spring equinox. Chinese time is forever tied to the twelve creatures who offered their farewells to the dying Buddha. These twelve fixed our years and hours to the stars and circling planets, patterning earthly time after cosmic time. The first of these sentient beings was the rat, who presides over the beginning of things and the hours marking midnight.

The year of the rat coincided with my eighth year. That rat presided over our family's move from Burbank to San Jose and the purchase of our first home in 1960. It watched as prune orchards were devoured and tract homes were developed for burgeoning boomer broods. It was the year I got saved at a hellfire-and-brimstone revival that scared the bejesus out of me.

After the Christmas ultimatum of 1971 my second rat year arrived with a second family and a second home. My first lover, Bruce, lived in a big Santa Barbara house with about four other guys and an ex-lover who became both father and mother to the lot of us. If anyone dared to poison my new home with violent words or deeds, I would just leave for the beach, the bar, or a trick's house. The second rat also brought my first job and my first introduction to the hospital. In both German and Norwegian the hospital is literally a sick house—*Krankenhaus, Sykehus.*

Twelve years later my third rat year arrived with a season of death and a home in which we would bear it. My best friend, Gabe, and I knew that gay lovers were likely to be transitory. We both wanted a real, lasting family, so we formed one with each other. A few years before Gabe and I had promised each other never to let careers or lovers separate us. We exchanged wedding bands to signify our commitment. In ancient times platonic love was even more highly regarded than sexual or romantic love, but only a few modern folk understood that we were neither lovers nor simply friends.

Physically Gabe was striking. Standing six feet, four inches tall and weighing 215 pounds, he had a commanding presence, even at the gym he attended religiously for over twenty years. His passions included all types of dance and as many types of men, and his massive muscles and devastating charm ensured that most people were passionate about him, too.

Gabe published numerous works on dance, including two histories of major American ballet companies. He once told me that truly great ballet transforms five fixed positions on the ground into seemingly effortless flying that can transcend the boundaries between heaven and earth. He was fascinated with the ambiguities of the human condition, as he revealed in a lecture he once gave on *Swan Lake* at Stanford University:

Even though you have seen *Swan Lake* dozens of times; even though you know precisely what happens and when it happens; even though you know how pointless it is to hope for another ending, doesn't a prayer still form on your lips? Doesn't your heart still swell with painful whispers that beg the prince not to betray his beloved for her tragic counterfeit? Don't we almost hope to touch his heart with the truth in our own? And then what happens? In one split second we are thundering with applause and shouting bravos at the Black Swan's dance of seduction. Such is the magic of theater. We not only see our ambiguities, we experience them.

Gabe loved dancers who flew through the heavens, but he wanted a domestic life that was rooted to the ground. Gabe thought we should start saving money for a down payment on a house. I thought that was impractical and would take way too long and suggested visualization and prayer. So we prayed for a home—twice, I think. God does not often speak to me in language that I clearly understand, but when I told Gabe that God had instructed me to engage a real estate agent, he agreed without an argument. After an evening of house hunting we'd often look at each other amazed and ask what we'd do if we actually found something we wanted. Neither of us had the money. The long and the short of it was that we got a rather unscrupulous partner whom we had to endure for a couple of years. The building was a wreck, but for almost no money down we bought one-third of a San Francisco Victorian and moved in on Halloween 1984—another rat year.

But my friends don't mark the 1980s and 1990s with Chinese animals, houses, or even AIDS discoveries. We mark out those decades with the deaths of our friends and loved ones.

1983—Mickey died.	1990—Ben died.
1985—Chuck died.	1991—Gabe died.
1986—Steve died.	1993—Jason died.
1987—Chris died. Duckus died.	1995—Dick died.
1989—Robert died.	

Death came of age, began flexing his muscles, showing his stuff, in 1983. We had perhaps given the Devil a bit more than his due, and he wreaked havoc with the surplus. Mickey's liver gave out first. He was

Steve's best friend's lover. Mickey had certainly consumed more drugs than the rest of us, and his doctor said it wasn't AIDS. For some reason Mickey was relieved. It made a difference to him. He was thirty-three.

Then in 1984 Jesse died. Chuck died in 1985. Steve died in 1986. Duckus died in 1987. One afternoon Gabe told his friend Toby about the four deaths that he and I had experienced together. Toby had known Gabe since he was a student at Stanford—longer than any of us. Fortunately, they decided to tape it. Gabe's retelling breathes some life back into those deaths. It illuminates what has come to be some of my own private darkness. It preserves a small piece of my family's and community's history.

▼▼▼

"The thirties is a time when people start coming to terms with getting older and mortality. Not that you're necessarily about to dig your grave or find your tombstone, but nevertheless, as you approach forty, you start dealing with mortality. But since this whole decade of my thirties has also coincided with AIDS, it's made the somewhat normal process of coming to terms with mortality that much more intense. Inescapably intense.

"Actually, the first person I ever saw dead was a person with AIDS. I came of age in an era in America where we shunted aside dead people. When I was growing up, there were no elderly grandparents around who were sick and then subsequently died. I'd never attended a funeral and certainly never touched a person who had died. Until Jesse. He died in 1984. One day I was supposed to go to the hospital because it was my shift, so to speak.[1] Instead, I got a phone call from Ernest, who was both Jesse's lover and the person whose shift directly preceded mine. So I wasn't surprised when Ernest called. I just thought he was going to say, 'Come early' or something. But I became surprised and shocked because he said, 'Jesse is dead. Could you come over and help?'

"I left work very agitated and met Ernest in the hallway before I realized—I mean, the many other issues aside and the many other emotions aside—I was going to have to go into the room and see Jesse dead, and I had never seen anyone dead before. There were many issues, needless to say—my own grief, my own concern for Jesse, my own concern for Ernest, and any number of other issues. But all of these were colored by the fact that all of a sudden I was going to do something I had never done, and I didn't know exactly how I was going to respond or react. I actually went in, and in my fashion—it's my fashion, so to speak, particularly in the presence of other people, to rise to the occasion.

"Richard was also at work, but he assured us that he would come as soon as possible, so that made things a lot easier. But until Richard got there, I thought it was my responsibility to help Ernest. I didn't know what I was doing, but I thought we were supposed to clean Jesse up a little bit because his mom was on her way from Florida.

"And Ernest wanted Jesse's ring and for some reason couldn't take the ring off, and I said I would. I did things like that. But my real response was very strange. Part of me was totally freaked out, but that part I kept to myself. The other part was, I don't want to say intellectual, but I was so curious and bewildered by what was going on. I've had a lot of sex in my life, and I've been next to a lot of men's bodies. I remember feeling him and touching him as he was getting colder, but the most strange thing was that there was no heartbeat. That was one of the most radically disturbing and intriguing moments of my life. All of a sudden, the very basic components of the human body were rent open. It's the most basic thing that you know about the human body. It flushes and it's warm and it beats. All of a sudden that basic premise no longer held, and at first I didn't know what to make of that. On the surface, I was doing things for Ernest, and I was helping Richard, and I was trying to take care of things. But at the end of a very long day when I was finally alone, when the reverberations of the event took over and I started to realize what had happened, what I had seen, and what I had done, I couldn't fully comprehend it.

"When I looked at Jesse, he didn't look happy after he was dead, and in my little cosmology, personal cosmology, if you couldn't be happy when you were dead, something was radically wrong. I went to a shrink for about six weeks after Jesse died. I had never gone to a shrink, unlike most of my friends, but I was experiencing some unhappiness. During those six weeks we found out that what was very disturbing for me was not that Jesse had died, although that was disturbing enough, but that he didn't look resolved, he didn't look happy afterwards."

▼ ▼ ▼

Nobody who dies on a respirator looks happy. As a nurse I didn't expect Jesse to look happy, even after the tubes were taken out. But Gabe's concern went deeper than I had initially understood. Gabe's first experience with death did not conform to the choreography he had composed in his mind. The space between heaven and earth was not transcended effortlessly, happily. The dancer was young and strong, but far from willing to make the leap. Gabe's cosmology had not yet incorporated the Catholic or Eastern customs of helping the dead along with prayers. He did not yet understand that many of us limp, rather than fly, into heaven. Yet despite all of Gabe's spiritual vision and sense of completion, despite all of his strength and emotional intelligence, on the day of his own death he looked neither willing nor happy. But within days of Gabe's death I am convinced that he was saying prayers for me.

▼ ▼ ▼

"So Jesse died in 1984 and Chuck died in 1985. I think Richard actually met Jesse through Chuck. And Chuck was an ex-lover of Steve, Richard's ex-lover. Chuck was one of those people I count as in-laws—you know, the people that we'd see at Thanksgiving, Christmas, parties, birthdays, and things. I think Chuck was actually interested in dating me, and although we never did, we liked each other a lot. We'd certainly been to a lot of parties together.

"Seeing Chuck was one of the great, weird moments in my life. I hadn't seen him much after he got sick, but the week he was dying, Richard asked me to go over to see whether I could help with things. And I remember looking in the room and saying to myself, I'm in the wrong house. That was my first thought. I'm in the wrong room. I couldn't see the Chuck that I knew there at all. I had to stop and catch my breath and look closely before I realized that it in fact was Chuck. It was like when we go see a horror movie or fantasy film and we think, oh, this is just ridiculous; this doesn't happen. But in some sense crazy things do happen in life. Seeing those physical changes in Chuck was like one of those sci-fi movie transformations. It was like a disappearing act, black magic. It had nothing to do with the Chuck who I knew in that very first instant. I mean, obviously, after a while your rational processes take over and you realize, oh, he's just lost a lot of weight or he's aged. But in that first instant it was like those movies where Jekyll becomes Hyde, the beast becomes the man, the frog becomes the prince. Some mythic, radical, dramatic, almost unfathomable transformation occurs. And I thought, I'm in the wrong house; how do I get out?

"Since then I've had similar experiences walking into hospital rooms. I would hear through friends that someone was sick and if you wanted to go see him, you should see him now, and he's in room 222. But when

I walked into room 222, I thought, oh, I must have walked into room 223 because I don't know this person. That's happened quite a bit.

"It sounds so awful, but it's disturbing how quickly you assimilate all this. I was there on Friday, and by the time I saw him dead on Saturday, his appearance didn't disturb me. There was actually a very clear progression. I saw Jesse after he was dead, but I didn't really take care of him that much when he was in the hospital. I took care of Jesse in other ways, like buying him food and helping him go shopping. I helped take care of Chuck when he was very sick, on the last day. And in just a few months after Chuck died, Steve got sick."

▼ ▼ ▼

By Christmas 1984 both Mickey and Jesse were dead and Chuck was already sick. None of us could quite comprehend it. Yet there was still Christmas to celebrate or to get through. Gabe's and my new house was still pretty much a mess, but we managed to get one of the double parlors together. The eleven-and-a-half-foot ceilings were high enough to contain my fantasy Christmas tree. My lover, Steve (and every other taste queen I knew), had dictated that gay Christmas trees be decked with small, tasteful white lights. The big 1950s colored lights from my childhood had to go, but they were replaced with a collection of satin jesters, sparkling jewels, and shimmering glass icicles. A few pine cone elves still winked mischievously as the wise men suggested ancient joys in distant futures.

This was the last year that Steve Richter would drop by and the second time I saw him cry. The first time occurred when his cat, Isidora, died. Not an ounce of airy-fairy doctrine had infected Steve's modern thinking. Life was ultimately a cruel joke, and death proved the fact. Yet by the time he mounted the thirty-nine steps to my flat, the tree's wintergreen spirit had penetrated his slightly breathless body to the bone. He was broken and sobbed like a little child, "The worst thing about death is there won't be any more Christmases." My own time for breaking down would come later. "I know far more about these things than you do, sweetheart, and I promise you it isn't so. I will always find a way to bring Christmas to you, in this world and the next, no matter where, no matter what."

Now I understand what happens to the tears a mother cannot allow herself to spill when comforting her own suffering child. They are deposited like coins in a wishing well. Every year I find that well suspended beneath some glistening bough and take the promised Christmas to him once again.

▼ ▼ ▼

This was how Gabe experienced Steve's illness: "I took care of Steve a lot physically when he was ill. He had chills and seizures, and I remember having to hold him when he was shaking. He was having lots of troubles, and I would actually get in bed with him to try to keep him warm or calm down his breathing or any number of things. I'm not a nurse, so I didn't do the physical applications, but a lot of the other kinds of things, from changing sheets to just holding him or hand-feeding him or bathing him by hand. Have you ever tried to get someone into a bathtub when they don't have their full capacities? Anyway, I did stuff like that.

"But Steve's situation was quite different from Jesse's and Chuck's. He was taken care of at home, so he required a lot of care. And he put up such a struggle! He had a major debilitating seizure and didn't die for almost five or six months. As far as I was concerned, he was kind of gone for most of that time.

"Although a lot of people thought that Steven and I were somewhat alike, after he had the seizure, I somewhat disassociated myself from that part of him. I couldn't imagine—I could be totally wrong; how do you know about these things?—but I couldn't imagine myself ever fighting like that, holding on like that. I think I would have just died. I thought he would have died, too, because I'm sure the Steven that I knew didn't want to have anything to do with the Steven that he turned into. He didn't have most of his capacities, and although he certainly enjoyed a few things, his great pleasures in life were no longer available to him as far as I could tell from my limited point of view. So it was kind of strange. Why was he holding on so long?"

▼ ▼ ▼

This question is a common question. Even though it can never be answered with certainty, we are nonetheless compelled to search for meaning in what we can barely comprehend. Steve was probably more fastened to this earth than most of us, yet I preferred to think that Steve was discovering how unconditionally he was loved. But Gabe's question wasn't as much about Steve as it was about what might happen to himself. Many people thought Gabe and Steve were "somewhat alike," and Gabe could not picture himself in the helpless and hopeless condition in which he saw Steve. As others have noted, we see our own death in the deaths of our loved ones, and Gabe's first three experiences with death were not easy mirrors in which to contemplate his own. When the time came, Gabe tried to hold on, too, although his body did not let him.

Chris Engelbach, our blond bombshell and fairy prince, was the next to die. His blue eyes were fractured with a light that could make the sea blush. When he smiled at me, I would drop soft kisses on the high cheekbones and broad brows that anchored his amazing eyes to this world. The last time, he was soaking up rays falling against the blistered wall of a Laundromat, a few pounds lighter, a bit drawn. My heart quickened and then dropped. There on that still-perfect face in the middle of the path my kisses had always taken stood a KS lesion. But even AIDS had difficulty damaging this creature. We spent a joyful afternoon in each other's arms. We may have cried. I don't remember. My kisses followed their predestined path.

Two weeks later I got a card from the Northwest where he was visiting his parents. I was moved that our afternoon together had been memorable enough for him to send a note. That was uncommon in my experience, no matter how pleasant the time may have been. What astonished me, however, was that he had ended it with a poem that went something like this:

> Some people walk into your life and quickly go,
> Others come and stay awhile, leaving footprints on your heart,
> And you are never, ever the same.

I had no idea that he wrote poetry. I tucked that card into the pocket of my calendar and carried it with me for over a year. Our sex together may have been casual, but our feelings for each other were far from shallow. I never saw him again.

Gabe had known him, too, of course. Gabe knew all of my boyfriends, lovers, and fairy princes, and he was as amazed at the poem as I was—and as saddened by Chris's death. But the most profound death in our lives together was Duckus's, and this is the story he told to Toby.

"As you know, I'm very much a home, a domestic person. So whereas watching Steve hang on for so long and seeing Jesse die in the hospital was disturbing, it was somewhat easier than when Duckus died. It was never easy, but when I came home, my home was still home. When Duckus was diagnosed, he actually lived with me in my flat because our other partner was still living upstairs with Richard. Duckus and I had a long history. I knew him both from the gym and as Richard's lover, so I had been used to eating dinner with him every night, and there was so much more emotional resonance. And his death was much faster.

"We knew that Duckus was going to die, and we brought him home about a week before. That whole week was very, very tumultuous for me. The day he died I could barely get out of bed, which is not like me at all. When I finally did, it was a very, very beautiful day. I was sitting in the living room with his mother and another friend of ours, Sharon. Richard knew the moment was close and somehow got the strength—I don't know how—to read him a meditation on dying from an author the two of them had studied. And Richard was about halfway through the meditation when Duckus sat straight up in bed because when we got into the room, he was sitting up. He actually started to die by sitting up.

"There was one slight moment where he took a breath back, and I thought he was going to struggle or fight a little bit to stay alive, but for the most part his eyes opened and his face was—I know this sounds clichéd, but his face was beatific, and his eyes opened and opened, and it looked like he was God, and he looked like the doors of heaven. I mean you could basically hear the music come on, and everything that you hold sacred about heaven, that kind of transcendence and transformation, that going on to a different plane, seemed utterly palpable on his face. To see that look. I mean, how could you feel sad when you were seeing death and transfiguration right in front of your face? How many times in life do you get to see that transfiguration, that powerful transformation right there in front of your eyes on a face you were very used to reading, you know, because I had known his face very well? And physically he was still very beautiful when he died.

"I had so many mixed emotions. Obviously, I started to cry right away, but everyone else was softly telling him to go for it. At first I had a little trouble with that because we have so many instincts to hold on. He wasn't in any pain. And Richard helped him to lie back down, and he put his hands on Duckus's head and asked me to put mine on his heart. And we all saw his eyes opening up and his eyes opening up more and his eyes opening up more and more and more and more as he was dying.

"There are moments in life, whether it's watching a movie or watching someone act or dance or sing, that human beings jump into the other person. You somehow identify with them to such an extent that you almost become them. At that moment I became Duckus. I always thought the phrase 'that a part of me died with him' meant something different. I always thought that the part of you that had fun, or a part of you that lived your life with that person, died. But when Duckus died, the phrase meant something totally different. 'A part of me died' was almost literally true. It seemed like I was dying as well, but not in a scary way because he didn't seem frightened.

"After he died, we ordered balloons and champagne and ate dinner in his room. We all did an incredible number of rituals with his body that day, including dressing him and bathing him and getting him ready, eventually ten hours later to be taken out. To this day I cannot believe that we had him for ten hours before the funeral home picked him up. I mean it just seems like, how could I have stayed in the house for ten hours, and what did I do? But the most relevant thing for me was that for many, many hours afterward I was high as a kite. I don't mean that literally. I wasn't on drugs or anything. But although there was an enormous sense of loss, and there were many, many emotions happening at once, the most powerful one was that I was high. It was such an intense experience that I was swept up in it. His energy so pervaded the house and the metaphysical reality of his being there one minute and his not being there the next—but his body still remaining—was so dizzying and electrifying that I felt intoxicated. It was much later, a day or so later, that the real pain started. But the day he died I was not in an enormous amount of pain. I was as much with him in whatever world he was in as I was in this world. This world had very little reality for me at that moment. I was swept away by where he could possibly be and tried to transport myself with him, knowing that I had full ability to come back."

▼▼▼

What Gabe didn't tell Toby was this: the day before Duckus died, I tried to think of whom I wanted to welcome him to heaven. When Steve died, the choice was easy. His good friend Mickey and his ex-lover

Chuck had preceded him, and I asked them both to greet him.

This isn't as glib as it might sound. My prayer was that if it was possible, if it made a difference, if it would not interfere with a better plan for Duckus, then I should like to ask that Chris, our fairy prince, meet him at the gate or the tunnel or whatever it was. Over the course of taking care of many dying people I had come to think of hospice nursing like obstetric nursing. The goal was to help smooth the transition from one totally different world to another. We put the baby's ear to the mother's chest so that it might take comfort from the familiarity of her heartbeat. Chris was the only soul I knew who might bridge the realms of earthly and heavenly love for Duckus. So I asked my angels to send Chris.

The next day the doorbell rang and a friend of a friend handed me some flowers and a card. The gay community in San Francisco was never big on sympathy cards, but I really appreciated this gesture. Upstairs I put the flowers in a vase and read the card:

Some people walk into your life and quickly go,
Others come and stay awhile, leaving footprints on your heart,
And you are never, ever the same.

Atheists and nihilists might dismiss our experience as a simple coincidence. As rational thinkers Gabe and I were only certain that Chris was not the poet. But as men who shared a similar cosmology, Gabe and I were certain that the spaces between heaven and earth are both inhabited and accessible, whether through dance or love or simply prayer.

▼▼▼

Gabe was used to taping what he thought might be momentous discussions. In 1980 he initiated two conversations with me that he also taped. So when I asked him if I could interview him for my dissertation research, he was already familiar with the process. As a writer and speaker, Gabe was an extremely articulate member of our community. Often it seemed as if he were delivering prepared texts, but this was not the case. Gabe thought in larger units than most people, in paragraphs rather than phrases.

We had our interview about HIV in his living room underneath a giant whimsical black-and-white portrait of Billie Holiday that Toby had painted. I sat on a modern white pillow couch while Gabe leaned his large body back into his black leather reading chair. Like Dick, Gabe was all class.

▼ ▼ ▼

"At what point did HIV start affecting your life?"

"With few exceptions, I don't think that there was a day when all of a sudden something was demarcated. It's been a far more gradual shift from one color into another. At first I thought that it was only hitting a particular fringe segment of the community. But then I realized that most likely I was included in that segment of the community which was infected with whatever disease it was. Mickey's illness and death was certainly one of those shifts. Something did shift at that time. He certainly partied more and he probably fucked more, but he was somebody I knew, so it had a kind of specificity and immediacy. He wasn't a close friend, but he was someone who traveled in my circle of friends.

It's almost been a decade now that we've been living with AIDS, and it's actually been very much a day-to-day thing. It's not a year-to-year thing. It's not a month-to-month thing. Maybe a few hours go by, but not a day goes by where I have not had to come to terms with some issue related to AIDS, either my own or a friend's. Sometimes it's specific things like going to the hospital to see somebody or wondering why I feel so tired or what this thing on my face is. Sometimes there are very large philosophical questions, like how does all of this relate to my whole life structure? I don't know when it's going to end, whether I'm included, how it will affect my friends, lovers, colleagues, coworkers, housemates. That changes your professional life, your romantic life, your sexual life, your emotional life, your spiritual life. All of a sudden it's like a new thread being woven into the fabric, and new colors and new patterns all of a sudden emerge. It's a very day-to-day thing. And over the days and years, as you can imagine, that's going to be a lot of changes.

"I have loved and embraced my community, and it has provided me with enormous support. But now my world has been devastated. I think it's very hard for people outside the situation to realize what it's like to live with the plague. Some people have the luxury of looking at AIDS on the cover of *Time* magazine or hearing about it from a distance. They can forget about it entirely for months or certainly weeks. Those of us who are HIV positive and those of us who live in cities like San Francisco don't have that luxury."

▼▼▼

Urban centers such as New York and San Francisco do offer several advantages for people living with HIV, but the luxury of not thinking about it is not one of them. Nathan noticed this after moving from Washington, D.C.; Jason noticed this after moving from Boston. Eric often told me that as a city San Francisco was infected with HIV—physically, emotionally, and socially. That's why Eric said he needed to escape it sometimes, even if it was just to the suburbs. Gabe discovered that luxury a few months after our conversation when he spent several days at Sea Ranch doing interviews for another documentary. When he returned, he remarked that it was strange and interesting to have been in a place where HIV was not all around.

But although Gabe noticed the difference, he didn't seek it. His world, though radically altered by HIV, was still clearly his world. Gabe's concept of his own body and his feelings about sex and men were also altered, but unlike Eric, he tended to struggle with the new metaphors and understanding, not against them.

Gabe's narrative also included an analysis of the gay community's new identity and sexuality and of how AIDS came to threaten both. But Gabe's account of the re-creation of the self through sex was different from those we have heard from Eric and Dick. For Eric, the dissolution and re-creation of the self were responses to oppressive male systems of power. For Dick, they were simply part of the joy of sex. For Gabe, the dissolution of the self was about adventure.

▼▼▼

"In the late '70s and early '80s gay men operated upon a certain set of assumptions. Like any community, most of our assumptions were not articulated, but nevertheless loomed so large that perhaps they now need to be articulated. One of those assumptions was that sex was healthy, literally and metaphorically. Another was that sex did not need to be monitored. Any kind of attempt to monitor or regulate it was viewed as a residue of Victorian repression or puritanical impulses.

"So here we were, one of the first generations (in America) and one of the first communities within that generation to fully embrace the sexual impulse. Sex was healthy and the human body was healthy. Then all of a sudden AIDS came along. It was like a bad play or a bad novel where the metaphor gets turned upside down. Sex was all of a sudden associated with disease—literally—as it had been historically. So the human body, as opposed to being this incredible vessel for pleasure and for exploration and adventure, all of a sudden became a vehicle for disease and death.

"For some good reasons, our culture followed a very conservative impulse, one that clearly favored stability. As a result, there were very few outlets in the late twentieth century for a middle-class person such as myself to explore the unknown, the exotic. Sex provided that outlet for my generation, especially for gay men. You could just plunge into the unknown, the exotic, and emerge differently, into new senses of self. The self was something to be created and reinvented. You went to the baths with a self that could be constructed, manipulated, altered, modified, right there on the spot. All of a sudden AIDS came along, and I don't mean to be crude, but it was no longer as adventuresome and no longer as fun. So that impulse, that arena of play, that arena of the dissolution of the self was lost to me for many, many years. And I mourn losing that sense of adventure as well as the deaths of my friends.

"To flip-flop, to reverse all of that in such a short time, was very, very difficult for me and for a lot of other people I talked to. I think any plague, any disease would be difficult for any community. But I think it was even harder for a community that had so clearly, powerfully, and persuasively identified the human body with pleasure and with sex, that had based its whole identity upon that sexual impulse.

"It's very hard sometimes to remember that we were the first generation to fully live in a postpenicillin world. If you read Shakespeare, love and sex are always alive with metaphors of disease, decay, and death. That's not only Shakespeare's sensibility. People had to be very careful about such diseases. When I came of age sexually, there were no questions about diseases. The floodgates just opened up in our generation because the sexual revolution of the '60s took place in a postpenicillin generation. I never even knew about the connection between sex and death because we had penicillin.

"On top of that, gay people did not even have to worry about birth control. In my world there was no history of monitoring the sexual impulse for any health or societal reasons. I was accustomed to indulging whatever I wanted to whenever I wanted to. And philosophically I associated that indulgence with a certain kind of liberation. When AIDS came along and reversed those associations, all of a sudden new associations, new metaphors, new imagery came along. It really has radically changed my sense of the body, my sense of the sexual impulse, and what sex is about.

"I'd been going to the gym for a long time and had a body that was very attractive and very much in demand, particularly in the late '70s. I had always seen myself as a sort of present to the world, and I could go out into that world and share that present, but in the AIDS world the body has become a vessel for disease. It was a radical change to think of my cock as an instrument of death instead of an instrument of pleasure. I'm very glad I know about condoms, and I certainly use them all the time. I've learned different tricks to do in order not to infect other people—like using condoms but still pulling out, even with a condom, prior to an orgasm. Nevertheless, the metaphor is far more powerful than the condom. Even when I'm taking precautions, the idea that I could be infecting someone has colored my own sense of my body and my dick, at least in some ways. At other times, to be honest, it's very hard to believe that the virus is in you because it's invisible, you know."

Gabe understood his sexuality as the "adventure" left open to the twentieth-century man, yet he posited adventure not as a social ideal, but as a necessary escape from the "conservative impulses" in society—impulses toward the hearth and family, impulses toward stable social identities and structures. Whereas these conservative impulses worked against the drive toward individuation and identity, Gabe did not vilify them. For Gabe, adventure was not about disrupting or challenging entrenched traditions or systems of power. Neither was it about isolationism or simple hedonism. Rather, adventure was what happened on the "hero's journey"—a metaphor I heard many times during our lives together.[2] The hero's journey always included leaving the hearth, undergoing hardship, confronting adversity, and discovering new worlds, new desires, and a new, more powerful self. The kingdom should be enriched by the hero's return, not revolutionized or destroyed. And the hero should return.

Gabe tended to confront the metaphors that linked sex and death within a context of historical narratives, cultural understandings, and personal experiences. Whereas some conceptualize history, epic, and narrative as structured systems of contemporary power, it was the essence and subject of myth and story that fascinated Gabe, not what they became under the sociological gaze.

Gabe characterized HIV as having changed his body from a vessel for pleasure into an instrument of death. Gabe incorporated the metaphors and shared social understandings that AIDS brought to the body politic. He recognized his own body as a potential instrument of death and implemented safe-sex practices from which he never deviated, but the body never lost its central value. Gabe had a long tradition of honoring the body, and he was emphatic that the body, and specifically his body, deserved respect.

Gabe had waited until 1989 to get his T cells checked, and I never quite understood the hesitation—except that, like Eric and Dick, he seemed resistant to "medicalizing" his life. Once during a conversation on another topic I abruptly asked him what the first thing was that came to his mind when he heard "AZT," and he said, "Death. Some people say 'Silence = Death.' For me, it has always been AZT = Death." I was concerned about Gabe's changing blood work and his initial reluctance to take AZT. Ultimately, Gabe decided to take AZT, and he had to struggle with his initial associations.

"There are two ways to approach something like AZT. One position treats the body as something that deserves to be poisoned. The other position appreciates that, for whatever reason, even though the body might be undergoing a siege, or undergoing a difficult time, that there are still other resources for the body and that the body deserves those other resources."

"What are those resources—things like vitamins or lifestyle changes?"

"As far as vitamins, alternative medicine, all that kind of stuff—no. That's not the level I operate on. Other people do, but that kind of stuff isn't congruent with the rest of my life. That's not the level at which my most important decisions take place, although I honor that level. I've never been particularly interested in support groups either, although I went to one for a while. For me, the whole community functions as a support group. In my case it was more about lifestyle changes. I've always been pretty good about sleep and things like that. And although I certainly took my fair share of drugs in the '70s, by the '80s I was already doing far less drugs, and now I do just about nothing.

"But honestly, things like diet and sleep and even drugs aren't on the level where my most important decisions take place either. No, with AIDS I just upped the dosage of something I have always been doing. Which is this: the really important thing is waking up in the morning and saying, 'This life makes sense to me. I like this life. What I do on a day-to-day basis, on a moment-to-moment basis, makes sense.' The rhythm, the way you dance to it makes sense. The texture, the fabric feels right. That issue should be as important to someone who has one day to live as someone who has one decade, one century. It doesn't change. That's one thing I've learned from AIDS and have been able to implement in my life. I've actually been fairly lucky most of my life to try to live it so it makes sense to me, but with AIDS there was that much more imperative, that much more cause to make it make sense. I don't mean intellectual sense, though."

It took me a while to understand that Gabe had his own ways of honoring his body. The level on which Gabe cared for himself was not about health care or therapies, whether allopathic, holistic, or otherwise. These were not the matters that were most interesting to him. I was able to talk him into taking AZT, in part because his culture and lifeworld did include Western medicine, at least as a distinct theoretical possibility. I was not able to talk him into anything else. This was hard for me because as beautiful as Gabe's approach was, I was afraid he was getting sick.

"I'm not a physical person in the sense of a million sports, but I've been a very healthy person. I've gone to the gym five days a week for the past twenty years, and I can still lift 450 pounds—more than anyone else I know. But all of a sudden, because I'm now somewhat anemic, I cannot run up the stairs. My legs just give out. It sounds like such a little thing compared to my friends who have undergone personality changes or lost their memory or their ability to walk. It doesn't sound very severe, but it is a radical identity change. It sounds silly, but since I started taking AZT, I'm no longer a person who can run up the stairs. And I'm actually a little nervous sometimes. The other night was the first time I fucked a lot since I've been on the AZT. I was a little nervous about whether I would get winded fucking. I didn't. It was really nice, but I was very nervous, wondering what would happen if I got winded fucking this guy. I've always thought of myself as virile and as a man with an excess of energy and sexual energy. And all of a sudden there is a part of me that is a little feeble. That's been a real shock.

"I think the biggest change in my life was finding that the future is no longer in infinite supply. Most people in their twenties and early thirties, and probably even in their forties and fifties, assume that delayed gratification is only a delay. We live so much of our lives in delayed gratification because of the assumption that gratification would eventually come—namely, in a future. By 1985 that was just taken away. It wasn't that I was clear that we were all going to die, but you couldn't count on a future.

"We base a huge number of decisions on what we might want to do ten years from now or fifteen years from now. Everything from buying a second home to if I take step 'A' in my career now, it will lead to steps 'B,' 'C,' and 'D'—all that kind of linear thinking. Once you took the first step away, the whole set of dominoes fell, for me and for a lot of my friends. So a lot of decisions simply disappeared with the future, and we focused on more mundane questions like what to do today, what to do next month, maybe what to do next year. But the lines that so naturally and so quickly extend out from our own narratives about ourselves, that extend out into the future—all those lines, all of a sudden were chopped, all of a sudden ended in an abrupt chasm. The lines didn't extend very far out into the future. They could go only from here to maybe tomorrow, from here maybe to next month.

"To be honest, I think far too much of our culture is about delayed gratification, about future tripping, about what could happen fifteen to twenty years from now. We don't live frequently enough in the present. We are interested in becoming, not being. In some sense I've been filled with being, and that was quite nice. I really did live more completely in the present. The downside is that the future is also quite a nice place. A certain amount of our lives is based on decisions way down the road, and it's fun to think about decisions way down the road sometimes. I don't think about it much anymore. It is harder sometimes. It's harder to do.

"These are some of the larger issues I sometimes have trouble articulating succinctly. I'm not the first person to say this, but even though

AIDS or any other life-threatening disease may initially seem like a deviation from the norm, it is actually the essence of the norm. Our lives are always about death. It isn't a question of if we are going to die, but when. Any life that is totally divorced from death or that denies death is not a life at all. Life has to be fueled by, informed by, and part-nered by death because that is the way of the world, the way of the flesh, and there is nothing inherently bad about it. It is unfortunate that there is pain and loss, but death is not a sin. That is one of the great les-sons that AIDS has taught me. Our culture tends to equate life with suc-cess and death with failure, and that is a terrible, terrible formulation, a terrible definition."

▼▼▼

We both agreed that death was not a failure and that our culture erred enormously in construing it as one. We had both read Norman O. Brown and Ernest Becker.[3] But if I could not save Gabe, the world I had some-how managed to retain would collapse utterly. Gabe was what was left of my world, and his being was so huge, his intellect so powerful, his soul so luminous that, except for not being my "lover," he could fill my world entirely. I could not yet face that I might lose him, too.

▼▼▼

"You didn't really ask political questions, like how I feel about the gov-ernment's response or how I treat this as a political creature or as a social creature as opposed to a personal one. I don't subscribe to some of ACT-UP's philosophies, and I'm not quite as angry because I never looked to the government for quick action. But I still am angry at the medical community because they did a great disservice to us. Each year they would come along and say now we think the average incubation period is five years, then six, seven, eight years. And maybe they are just trying to cover their own asses and being safe and coming up with the most dire figures, the darkest predictions. But they never realized how those predictions would function in the community. Not that they should censor those predictions. But I thought the predictions about how long it would take before an HIV-positive person would develop AIDS were stupid, and I thought that years ago.

"And also the percentage of HIV-positive people who would suppos-edly go on to develop AIDS. By October of '89 we started hearing that no longer is it going to be 100 percent, but that wasn't what we heard for years and years. That was my belief years ago, though medicine is not my field. I've never heard of a virus moving through a population in a single, consistent, monolithic fashion. Namely, that it kills everybody. I always thought there would be a spectrum, a continuum. It may not be a simple bell-shaped curve, but I always thought that it would move through a population in different ways. It seemed evident that that was the case. Some of my friends were being infected and dying in two years. Others were being infected and getting sick eight years later. Some were being infected and not getting sick at all nine years later. So obviously there were other co-factors that the virus was coexisting in bodies in different ways. That does not mean I am unduly optimistic about everyone. But I thought that the medical community should have recognized that first and foremost. The medical community never seemed to acknowledge that. Now finally, years later, we are hearing doctors say, 'Oh, by the way, more people might survive than we thought. The nineties might not be what we predicted.' I thought that was unconscionable. I'm actually much prouder of what the gay community did than what the medical community did.

"I think, both as a writer and a person who loves narratives and myths and legends, that it is incredibly important to always generate some narrative, some scenario, in which there is somebody who survives, where there is some outcome that makes sense. Because without it, if you really did believe five years ago that it was 100 percent and everyone was going to die, how could you possibly ever look for alternatives, whether it be AZT or acupuncture or herbs? Whether I survive or not is not the relevant thing. Unless there is some scenario in your mind, some narrative, some dramatic line in which your community will survive and someone will overcome the virus, then there is no possibility of overcoming the virus. You have already said the virus is stronger than your community. Whether I am the one who is the character in that scenario who survives isn't the most relevant thing, but the fact that the scenario is there. I actually feel proud of our community because over the years we looked for different scenarios. Whether it was ddI or drugs—some of which didn't work out—that is not the relevant thing: people looked for scenarios. People looked for narratives in which someone would triumph, in which someone would win, in which someone, if for no other reason, would be there to chronicle and pay witness to that majority of us who were dying.

| 10 |

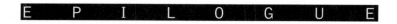

This study was not aimed at discovering universals. Just as blood cannot be transfused from every body to every body, the meanings uncovered through narrative research cannot be generalized to populations. Like blood types, however, some stories contain patterns or themes that can be taken up or incorporated into another person's life. Narratives are not taken up in the totality that one may absorb the blood of another, but are more often partially incorporated. Even those stories that are too foreign to be of practical value in our own lives can function like fiber in the diet, not absorbed perhaps but appreciated in other ways. Stories can help us to differentiate between ourselves and others. They can also help us to loosen fixations and facilitate an appreciation for a wide variety of possibilities within the world.

Neither is the fundamental purpose of narrative research to discover and manipulate variables in order to produce desired changes. Rather, the purpose is, as Florence Nightingale said, to put the patient in an environment where nature can do its work.[1] Nature heals best when people are in environments that sustain hope, possibility, and meaning. People heal best when those environments help them retain their essential humanity in the face of challenges, suffering, and loss. Healing environments cannot flourish without diversity, without art, without narrative, without the humanities. It isn't enough for nurses and physicians to see the patient behind the disease—at least not at the price this country is paying for health care. We need to make understanding our patients a much higher priority, and that can't happen unless we respect and listen to them.

This research did not tell me the secret of surviving with asymptomatic HIV. It did not demonstrate the superiority of one health ideology or practice over another. I still don't know if we should all be taking the cocktail or not. I still don't know if unprotected sex between two HIV-positive lovers is okay or not. But neither does anyone else, despite the proliferation of national guidelines and recommendations that encourage us to take drugs and avoid Caesar salads.

I did learn that not everyone thinks these are the central issues. Even my best friend did not seem interested. Yet as a nurse I still wonder how many of the thirty-odd diseases we call AIDS are due to HIV and how many are due to these vague phenomena called co-factors. I still wonder whether it was HIV that caused Steve's progressive multifocal leukoencephelopathy or his cocaine use. I still wonder whether it was HIV that caused Jason's wasting syndrome or the fact that the hundredth monkey hadn't figured out HIV was a manageable condition yet. I still wonder whether it was HIV that caused Duckus's pneumocystis pneumonia or the poppers that he did before we got together. I still wonder whether it was HIV that caused Gabe's cryptosporidium or the AZT that I talked him into taking.

Sometimes I ask my friends on the other side what it was primarily that caused their early deaths: "Was it (a) HIV, (b) drugs, or (c) negative thinking?" I ask.

And all they ever do is smile and say, "You know how to take multiple-choice tests."

NOTES

Chapter 1. Before Cocktails

1. T-helper cells, or CD4 lymphocytes, are a subset of T cells. People commonly use the broader term *T cells* when speaking of CD4 cells.

2. See David Ho, A. U. Neuman, A. S. Perelson et al., "Rapid Turnover of Plasma Virions and CD4 Lymphocytes in HIV-1 Infection," *Nature* 373 (January 12, 1995): 123–126.

3. Burroughs Wellcome Co., "New Perspectives on HIV Pathogenesis," *Journal of the Association of Nurses in AIDS Care* 6(3) (1995): 8–9.

4. Leaders such as Arnold Relman, editor of the *New England Journal of Medicine*, have been calling for more research into the efficacy of our new medical technologies for nearly two decades.

For a discussion of evaluating technology in medicine, see Arnold Relman, "The New Medical-Industrial Complex," *New England Journal of Medicine* 303(17) (1980): 963–970. By 1993 there was well-designed scientific research on AZT that cast serious doubt on the wisdom of using it to treat everyone with asymptomatic HIV.

For final results of this study, see Concorde Coordinating Committee, "Concorde: MRC/ANRS Randomized Double-Blind Controlled Trial of Immediate and Deferred Zidovudine in Symptom-Free HIV Infection," *Lancet* 343(8902) (April 9, 1994): 871–881.

For a discussion of how these results were received in the United States, see Elinor Burkett, *The Gravest Show on Earth: America in the Age of AIDS* (Boston: Houghton Mifflin, 1995).

5. For early epidemiological research and projections, see Ron Brookmeyer, Gail Mitchell, and Frank Polk, "The Prevalent Cohort Study and the Acquired Immunodeficiency Syndrome," *American Journal of Epidemiology* 126(1) (1987): 14–24; John Fahey, Jeremy Taylor, Elizabeth Korns et al., "Diagnostic and Prognostic Factors in AIDS," *Mount Sinai Journal of Medicine* 53 (1986): 657–663; Gail Mitchell and Ron Brookmeyer, "Methods for Projecting Course of Acquired Immunodeficiency Syndrome Epidemic," *Journal of the National Cancer Institute* 80(12) (1988): 900–911; Nancy Hessol, Alan Lifson, Paul O'Malley et al., "Prevalence, Incidence, and Progression of Human Immunodeficiency Virus in Homosexual and Bisexual Men in Hepatitis B Vaccine Trials, 1978–1988,"

American Journal of Epidemiology 130(6) (1990): 1167–1175; Nancy Hessol, George Rutherford, and Paul O'Malley, "The Natural History of Human Immunodeficiency Virus Infection in a Cohort of Homosexual and Bisexual Men: A Seven-Year Prospective Study" (Paper presented at the Third International Conference on AIDS, Washington, D.C., 1987); William Heyward and James Curran, "The Epidemiology of AIDS in the U.S.," *Scientific American* 259(4) (1988): 72–81; George Lemp, Susan Payne, George Rutherford et al., "Projections of AIDS Morbidity and Mortality in San Francisco," *JAMA* 263(11) (1990): 1497–1501; Lui Kung-Jong, William Darrow, and George Rutherford, "A Model-Based Estimate of the Mean Incubation Period for AIDS in Homosexual Men," *Science* 240(4857) (1988): 1333–1335; Jonathan Mann, James Chin, Peter Piot et al., "The International Epidemiology of AIDS," *Scientific American* 259(4) (1988): 82–89; A. R. Moss, "Predicting Who Will Progress to AIDS," *British Medical Journal* 297 (1988): 1067–1068; A. R. Moss, P. Bacchetti, D. Osmond et al., "Seropositivity for HIV and the Development of AIDS or AIDS-Related Condition: Three-Year Follow-up of the San Francisco General Hospital Cohort," *British Medical Journal* 296 (1988): 745–750.

6. Janice Swanson, Carole Chenitz, Marianne Zalar et al., "A Critical Review of Human Immunodeficiency Virus Infection and Acquired Immunodeficiency Syndrome–Related Research: The Knowledge, Attitudes, and Practice of Nurses," *Journal of Professional Nursing* 6(6) (1990): 341–355.

7. Normal is generally defined as 400–1600, but most often people with HIV interpret 500 and even 800 as low. HIV-positive people usually have other abnormalities in their T-cell counts besides the absolute number of CD4 cells (such as the percentage of CD4 cells to total lymphocytes and the ratio of CD4 to CD8 cells).

8. Thrush and hairy leukoplakia are two opportunistic infections of the mouth that are often relatively minor.

9. Today even some physicians are distinguishing between 30,000 and 50,000, but this may have less to do with hard science than it does with prevailing theories and clinical goals that seek to reduce everyone's viral burden to zero.

10. See Peter Duesberg, *Inventing the AIDS Virus* (Washington, D.C.: Regnery, 1996). Duesberg's comments on protease inhibitors were presented at the University of Tromsø, April 10, 1997. See also Neville Hodgkinson, *AIDS: The Failure of Contemporary Science* (London: Fourth Estate, 1996). Duesberg does not accept Hodgkinson's notion that HIV does not exist, but Duesberg does assert that HIV is not pathological. Other critics maintain that HIV is pathological but assert that other factors contribute to the progression from asymptomatic HIV infection to AIDS.

11. "AIDS Deaths Drop Significantly for First Time," *Wall Street Journal,* February 28, 1997, B1–2.

12. Thomas McKeown, "Determinants of Health," in *The Nation's Health*, ed. Phillip Lee, Carroll Estes, and Nancy Ramsay, 2d ed. (San Francisco: Boyd and Fraser, 1984), 8.

13. Michael Callen, *Surviving AIDS* (New York: HarperCollins, 1990).

14. Rothenberg, cited in ibid., 39.

15. The only factor shared by a majority of Callen's survivors was a decision to reject the recommendation to take AZT, and later controlled studies seemed to substantiate Callen's findings. But the serious problems associated with AZT were not what made Callen's work unique. Callen's book said something even more important. The stories he told were like a portrait gallery of hope—a gallery where survival was depicted in a variety of poses, attitudes, and approaches. Those who understand life as turning exclusively on genes and microbes (and therefore chance alone) might conclude that Callen's survivors all shared a gene or a weaker strain of virus. I was never sure why some lived while others died, but for me they stood as icons of possibility and a community of hope.

16. Twenty years are not intended to imply an outside limit. Some men who participated in an old hepatitis research study in San Francisco were found to be HIV positive in 1978. Therefore, the longest-known amount of time that anyone has survived with HIV will be twenty-one years in 1999, twenty-two years in 2000, and so forth until every person who was HIV positive in 1978 is dead. At that point those who were positive in 1979 and 1980 must be followed until all of them are dead. Even then it would be hard to make a very good estimate because to do so would imply that the very first group to become infected was similar to the group infected later. This has not deterred some very successful academics from making such claims or newspapers from publishing them.

17. For a discussion and review of the literature on complementary and alternative medicine and HIV/AIDS, see Richard MacIntyre, William Holzemer, and Marianna Philipek, "Complementary and Alternative Medicine in HIV/AIDS: Part I: Issues and Context," *Journal of the Association of Nurses in AIDS Care* 8(1) (1997): 23–31; Richard MacIntyre and William Holzemer, "Complementary and Alternative Medicine in HIV/AIDS: Part II: A Literature Review," *Journal of the Association of Nurses in AIDS Care* 8(2) (1997): 25–38.

18. Those who hold the position that AIDS is the scourge of an angry God rarely consider that God must therefore be happiest with lesbians as their incidence of AIDS is significantly lower than that of heterosexuals.

19. I feel compelled to reiterate my general belief in the "HIV is the cause of AIDS" equation. To not believe in this scientific equation is to risk being dismissed as a crackpot. However, people with HIV felt compelled to carry banners stating, "HIV DOES NOT EQUAL AIDS," even before the advent of effective antiviral treatments. Even though many of the redhats at the NIH have come to accept the existence of co-factors—of other variables in the equation—they seem to prefer that these variables remain nameless. "HIV = AIDS" is a better slogan for the industry.

20. Gabriel Rotello, *Sexual Ecology: AIDS and the Destiny of Gay Men* (New York: Dutton, 1996).

21. Duesberg, *Inventing the AIDS Virus.*

22. Ibid.

23. See Michel Foucault, *Power/Knowledge: Selected Interviews and Other Writings, 1972–1977* (New York: Pantheon, 1980).

24. For a full discussion of the theoretical framework and methods that were used in this study, see chapters 1 and 2 of my dissertation, "Sex, Drugs, and T-Cells:

Symbolic Meanings Among Gay Men with Asymptomatic HIV Infection." Copies of dissertations are available through UMI, 300 N. Zeeb Rd, Ann Arbor, MI 48106. Phone numbers: 1-800-521-0600 and 313-761-4700. Order number: 9406617.

The primary theory and methods texts that guided the study were Patricia Benner and Judith Wrubel, *The Primacy of Caring: Stress and Coping in Health and Illness* (New York: Addison-Wesley, 1988); Nancy Burns, "Standards for Qualitative Research," *Nursing Science Quarterly* (1989): 44–52; Margaret Dunlap, "Shaping Nursing Knowledge: An Interpretative Analysis of Curriculum Documents from NSW Australia" (Ph.D. diss., University of California, San Francisco, 1990); Clifford Geertz, "Deep Play: Notes on the Balinese Cockfight," in *Interpretive Social Science: A Second Look,* ed. Paul Rabinow and William M. Sullivan (Berkeley and Los Angeles: University of California Press, 1987), 195–240; Clifford Geertz, "From the Native's Point of View: On the Nature of Anthropological Understanding," in *Interpretive Social Science: A Reader,* ed. Paul Rabinow and William M. Sullivan (Berkeley and Los Angeles: University of California Press, 1979), 225–241; Jürgen Habermas, *Knowledge and Human Interests,* trans. Jeremy J. Shapiro (Boston: Beacon Press, 1971); Martin Heidegger, *Being and Time,* trans. John Macquarrie and Edward Robinson, 7th ed. (New York: Harper and Row, 1962); Martin Heidegger, *The Basic Problems of Phenomenology,* trans. Albert Hofstadter, 2d ed. (Bloomington: Indiana University Press, 1982); Patricia Munhall and Carolyn Oiler, *Nursing Research: A Qualitative Perspective* (Norwalk, Conn.: Appleton-Century-Crofts, 1986); Martin Packer and Richard B. Addison, eds., *Entering the Circle: Hermeneutic Investigation in Psychology* (Albany: State University of New York Press, 1989); Paul Rabinow and William M. Sullivan, eds., *The Interpretive Turn: A Second Look,* 2d ed. (Berkeley and Los Angeles: University of California Press, 1987); Charles Taylor, *Human Agency and Language: Philosophical Papers,* vols. 1 and 2 (Cambridge: Cambridge University Press, 1985); Charles Taylor, *Sources of the Self* (Cambridge, Mass.: Harvard University Press, 1989); Max Van Manen, *Researching Lived Experience: Human Science for an Action-Sensitive Pedagogy* (Albany: State University of New York Press, 1990).

Chapter 2. Born Again

1. "Nelly" means effeminate.

2. This is a test involving the injection of radioactive dye to visualize the blood vessels in the brain.

3. Emmanuel Dreuilhe, *Mortal Embrace: Living with AIDS,* trans. L. Coverdale (New York: Hill and Wang, 1988).

Chapter 3. Fear and Trembling

1. The "ratio" refers to a ratio between CD4 and CD8 cells (or the T-helper and T-suppressor cells). The "percent" refers to the percentage of CD4 cells to all the lymphocytes, including the CD8 and other lymphocytes.

2. Louise Hay is a leading advocate of self-healing through love. She wrote books and made inspirational tapes that have been popular among some holistic health enthusiasts and among many people confronting life-threatening illnesses. Like many approaches, Louise Hay's material can either empower or provoke unrealistic expectations of personal responsibility and guilt.

3. This egg lecithin product was supposed to make the walls of the blood cells more slippery, thus making it more difficult for the virus to attach and penetrate. Duckus and I had done AL-721. When he died, I stopped taking it. Later I read a review of a study that concluded that AL-721 reduced night sweats and the incidence of thrush but did nothing for the immune system. I remember being incensed. Science is still relatively ignorant concerning matters of the immune system, so to say what does and does not affect it at this point cannot possibly be well substantiated. The review was obviously substituting CD4 cells for the entire immune system. But despite dismissing the study results intellectually, I never took AL-721 again.

4. Supervision is the means by which psychiatric residents review issues related to their patients' therapy with the faculty psychiatrist who is overseeing their work.

5. Pentamidine is a drug used to prevent pneumocystis, one of the most prevalent and devastating opportunistic infections.

6. Neutrophils are white blood cells, and AZT depresses the bone marrow, where neutrophils are produced.

Chapter 4. Forecasts of Doom

1. Robert Root-Bernstein, *Rethinking AIDS: The Tragic Cost of Premature Consensus* (New York: Free Press, 1993); D. Hopkins, "Dr. Joseph Sonnabend," *Interview* Magazine (December 1992): 124–125, 142–143; Peter Duesberg, *Inventing the AIDS Virus* (Washington, D.C.: Regnery, 1996).

2. Early in the epidemic Kaposi's sarcoma was one of the leading causes of AIDS death among gay men. That this cancer has been rare to nonexistent among people with AIDS who are not gay has led some to question whether other factors besides HIV may be contributing to some KS and other AIDS diagnoses.

3. David M. Eisenberg, Ronald C. Kessler, Cindy Foster et al., "Unconventional Medicine in the United States," *New England Journal of Medicine* 328(4) (1993): 246–252.

4. Several people in my community sought to avoid sunburn, poison oak, and herpes outbreaks because these had been associated with increased viral replication in the gay press.

5. DdI was the second antiviral drug approved for HIV.

6. Lazarus was a popular disembodied spirit channeled by a clairvoyant. Lazarus gave people advice on health and other matters. Lazarus tapes and books were for sale in many urban gay neighborhoods. San Francisco's Castro district even had a Lazarus store.

Chapter 5. Two Friends

1. This was not really the case. It never became standard practice to give AZT to people with fewer than 400 T cells, although some physicians did prescribe AZT at even higher T-cell levels. By 1997 it was standard practice to treat everyone with antivirals regardless of T-cell count or viral load, but that was after a variety of antivirals became available. Even then there was serious disagreement concerning the advisability of treating asymptomatics with the cocktail. What is interesting here is that Ron perceived his own experimental treatment as an early instance of standard practice.

2. Concorde Coordinating Committee, "Concorde: MRC/ANRS Randomized Double-Blind Controlled Trial of Immediate and Deferred Zidovudine in Symptom-Free HIV Infection," *Lancet* 343(8902) (April 9, 1994): 871–881.

Chapter 6. Two Heretics

1. The riots in response to police raids at the Stonewall bar in New York marked the beginning of gay liberation in the United States.

2. This should not be surprising. The Robert Wood Johnson Foundation reported that physicians found it impossible to believe that middle-class white folks with signed living wills really preferred to die without life support and heroic treatment. Whether as a result of ignorance, arrogance, or both, those written directives were ignored as frequently as they were honored. But whenever values of patients are misunderstood or ignored, particularly the values of those whose age, sexuality, religion, and ethnicity are different from those of the health provider, the possibilities for rendering effective health care are seriously compromised. See Alfred Connors, Neal Dawson, Norman Desbiens et al., "A Controlled Trial to Improve Care for Seriously Ill Hospitalized Patients," *JAMA* 274(20) (1995): 1591–1598.

3. Like heterosexuals, many gay men use sex as an arena to enact fantasies or play roles that can attenuate unpleasant, traumatic, or humiliating experiences by eroticizing them. Sex can also be an arena where previous beliefs or notions about gender and identity are abandoned or reformulated.

4. This was a lubricant that had been identified as an excellent medium for parasites and came in a wide-mouthed container instead of a squeeze tube or pump bottle.

5. Along with typical sexually transmitted diseases, these included hepatitis, anal warts, and several varieties of intestinal parasites.

6. ACT-UP had demonstrated for quicker and cheaper access to AZT. Burroughs Wellcome, the pharmaceutical company that markets AZT, is now Galaxo Wellcome.

7. San Francisco General Hospital now offers people who had unprotected sex a "morning after" cocktail even before ascertaining if the patient contracted HIV. When liberal social ideals converge with powerful economic interests, the resultant political force is almost too powerful to stop, despite the fact that the vast majority of social liberals and academics seem to oppose the practice. It is as if we have

learned nothing at all from the well-documented dangers attending the inappro-priate use of antimicrobial agents. See Leslie Garret, *The Coming Plague: Newly Emerging Diseases in a World Out of Balance* (New York: Farrar, Straus and Giroux, 1994).

8. Sigmund Freud, *Totem and Taboo,* trans. A. A. Brill (New York: Vintage Books, 1946); Norman O. Brown, *Life against Death: The Psychoanalytic Meaning of History,* 2d ed. (Middletown, Conn.: Wesleyan University Press, 1985); Ernest Becker, *The Denial of Death* (New York: Free Press, 1973); Simon Watney, *Policing Desire: Pornography, AIDS, and the Media* (Minneapolis: University of Minnesota Press, 1987).

Chapter 7. Fire Island

1. The p24 is one of HIV's proteins or antigens. In 1990 a positive antigen indi-cated viral activity, but a negative p24 antigen meant very little, as many people with full-blown AIDS had negative p24 antigens.

2. In some circumstances unsafe sex may be less related to passions of the moment than to rational decisions that weigh risks against benefits. See S. Pinkerton and P. Abramson, "Is Risky Sex Rational?" *Journal of Sex Research* 29(4) (1992): 561–568; C. Donovan, C. Mearns, R. McEwan et al., "A Review of the HIV-Related Behavior of Gay Men and Men Who Have Sex with Men," *AIDS Care* 6(5) (1994): 605–617; J. McLean, M. Boulton, M. Brookes et al., "Regular Partners and Risky Behavior: Why Do Gay Men Have Unprotected Intercourse?" *AIDS Care* 6(3) (1994): 331–341.

3. See Michel Foucault, *The History of Sexuality,* Vol. 1, *An Introduction,* trans. Robert Hurley (London: Penguin, 1979), 95–96.

Chapter 8. The Agnostic

1. Søren Kierkegaard, *Either/Or,* trans. Howard Hong and Edna Hong, vol. 2 (Princeton, N.J.: Princeton University Press, 1987).

2. Søren Kierkegaard, *The Sickness unto Death,* trans. Howard Hong and Edna Hong (Princeton, N.J.: Princeton University Press, 1983); Sigmund Freud, *Mourning and Melancholia,* in *A General Selection from the Works of Sigmund Freud,* ed. John Rickman (Garden City, N.Y.: Anchor Books, 1937); Ernest Becker, *The Denial of Death* (New York: Free Press, 1973); Ken Wilbur, *Up from Eden: A Transpersonal View of Human Evolution* (Boston: Shambhala, 1986).

3. "Eighth and Howard" and "Rich Street" were gay bathhouses where one could find a variety of partners and spaces, including public areas for group sex and tiny private rooms for more intimate sex.

4. As a firm believer in condoms I kept encouraging Dick to consider them. I particularly recommended the natural skin variety that some well-meaning social engineers wanted to outlaw because some viral particles might slip through the pores. My argument was that far fewer would slip through than with no condom at all. Natural skin condoms don't break down with the old oil-based lubricants

that our community had become accustomed to and that the public health officials were against. Oil-based lubricants tend to disintegrate the preferred latex variety condom, which often breaks during anal sex despite the user's following directions to the letter. My recommendation was to continue avoiding ejaculation inside but to try natural skin condoms and oil-based lubricants rather than abandon condoms altogether, but even this recommendation would not really work for Dick. He agreed that he might eventually manage condoms with "more practice," but if more practice meant more partners, other risks would increase.

Chapter 9. Heaven's Gate

1. Jesse was a nurse, and many of his friends were nurses. These particular nurses were reluctant to leave their loved ones in the care of professional strangers, even in a nice private hospital. We scheduled "shifts" for all of his closest friends so that he would never be alone.

2. See Joseph Campbell, *The Hero with a Thousand Faces* (Cleveland: World Publishing, 1949).

3. Norman O. Brown, *Life against Death: The Psychoanalytical Meaning of History*, 2d ed. (Middletown, Conn.: Wesleyan University Press, 1985); Ernest Becker, *The Denial of Death* (New York: Free Press, 1973).

Chapter 10. Epilogue

1. Florence Nightingale, *Cassandra* (Old Westbury, N.Y.: Feminist Press, 1979).

INDEX

ABOUT THE AUTHOR

Richard MacIntyre has been a registered nurse since 1975. He holds nursing degrees from Santa Barbara City College and California State University, Sacramento, and an M.S. and a Ph.D. in nursing from the University of California, San Francisco. He completed a postdoctoral fellowship at the International Center for AIDS Research and Clinical Training in Nursing, a World Health Organization affiliate at the University of California, San Francisco. He was the 1996–1997 Fulbright professor in nursing at the University of Tromsø, Norway. Dr. MacIntyre is currently an associate professor and chair of the Division of Health Sciences and the Department of Nursing at Mercy College in Dobbs Ferry, New York.